T0041874

PSORIASIS COOKBOOK + MEAL PLAN

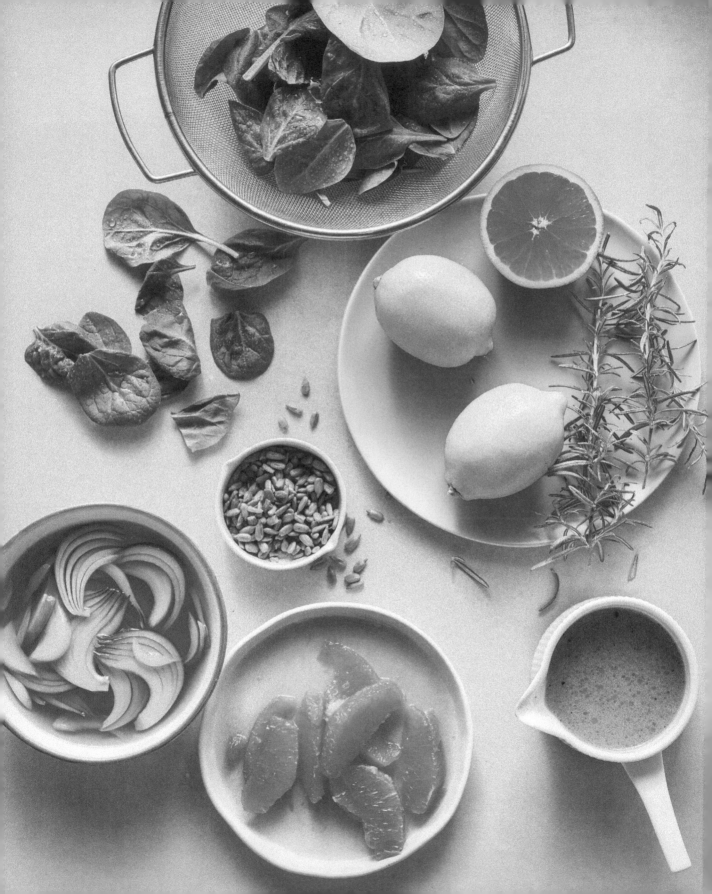

PSORIASIS COOKBOOK + MEAL PLAN

A Complete Guide to Relief with 75 Anti-Inflammatory Recipes

Kellie Blake, RDN, LD, IFNCP

ROCKRIDGE PRESS

Copyright © 2021 by Rockridge Press, Emeryville, California

No part of this publication may be reproduced, stored in a retrieval system, or transmitted in any form or by any means, electronic, mechanical, photocopying, recording, scanning, or otherwise, except as permitted under Sections 107 or 108 of the 1976 United States Copyright Act, without the prior written permission of the Publisher. Requests to the Publisher for permission should be addressed to the Permissions Department, Rockridge Press, 6005 Shellmound Street, Suite 175, Emeryville, CA 94608.

Limit of Liability/Disclaimer of Warranty: The Publisher and the author make no representations or warranties with respect to the accuracy or completeness of the contents of this work and specifically disclaim all warranties, including without limitation warranties of fitness for a particular purpose. No warranty may be created or extended by sales or promotional materials. The advice and strategies contained herein may not be suitable for every situation. This work is sold with the understanding that the Publisher is not engaged in rendering medical, legal, or other professional advice or services. If professional assistance is required, the services of a competent professional person should be sought. Neither the Publisher nor the author shall be liable for damages arising herefrom. The fact that an individual, organization, or website is referred to in this work as a citation and/or potential source of further information does not mean that the author or the Publisher endorses the information the individual, organization, or website may provide or recommendations they/it may make. Further, readers should be aware that websites listed in this work may have changed or disappeared between when this work was written and when it is read.

For general information on our other products and services or to obtain technical support, please contact our Customer Care Department within the United States at (866) 744-2665, or outside the United States at (510) 253-0500.

Rockridge Press publishes its books in a variety of electronic and print formats. Some content that appears in print may not be available in electronic books, and vice versa.

TRADEMARKS: Rockridge Press and the Rockridge Press logo are trademarks or registered trademarks of Callisto Media Inc. and/or its affiliates, in the United States and other countries, and may not be used without written permission. All other trademarks are the property of their respective owners. Rockridge Press is not associated with any product or vendor mentioned in this book.

Interior and Cover Designer: Mando Daniel
Art Producer: Sara Feinstein
Editor: Annie Choi
Production Editor: Matthew Burnett
Production Manager: Michael Kay

Cover Photography © 2021 Hélène Dujardin. Food styling by Anna Hampton. Interior photography © Antonis Achilleos, p. ii, 4; Emulsion Studio, p. vi, 38-39; Hélène Dujardin, p. 1, 12; Andrew Purcell, p. 24, 72, 108; Thomas J. Story, pps. 2-3, 134; Stocksy/Nataša Mandić, p. 40; Annie Martin, p. 54; Nadine Greeff, p. 90; Darren Muir, p. 120.

Author photograph courtesy of Kimberly Gillmeister.

Cover: Mediterranean Tuna Salad, p. 74.

Paperback ISBN: 978-1-648-76869-9
eBook ISBN: 978-1-648-76870-5

R0

To all the wonderful women in my life who have taught me the importance of cooking for family. Especially my aunt, Dee-Dee Skeens, who always had fresh, wholesome food at the ready! And to my husband, Will, who will eat anything I cook, even when it doesn't turn out so great.

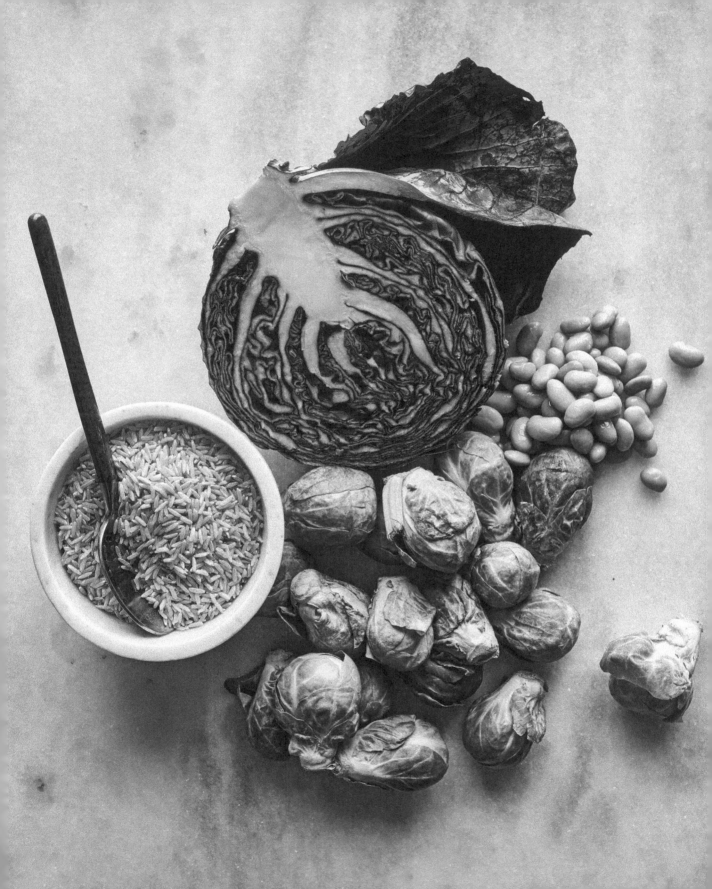

CONTENTS

INTRODUCTION

I was first diagnosed with psoriasis when I was 12 or 13 years old, but my symptoms began much earlier. I remember going to the doctor at the age of five and having my skin scraped onto a slide for review under a microscope. The doctor thought it was a fungal infection, but no treatment was offered and the area eventually cleared.

I continued to have skin symptoms, but it wasn't until my early teens that a dermatologist gave my symptoms a name: psoriasis. I was treated with topical steroids, creams, and shampoos, which provided some relief, but my symptoms always returned. My psoriasis plaques were located on my scalp—hidden from the rest of the world—until my early 20s, when they began to spread to the side and back of my neck, becoming more visible. Along with the physical discomforts, I now had to deal with the mental and emotional burdens that often accompany psoriasis.

My skin psoriasis has been in remission since my early 20s, but around that same time, I began experiencing more concerning autoimmune symptoms. I battled mouth sores, digestive issues, daily headaches, muscle and joint aches, lower back pain, interrupted sleep, swollen joints, and extreme fatigue. After years of seeing medical specialists and taking a variety of medications, I learned about nutrition and lifestyle medicine. I discovered how food affected my symptoms and how to make changes to my diet and lifestyle to target the root causes of my psoriasis and psoriatic arthritis symptoms. I no longer experience any of those worrisome symptoms, I take no prescription medication, and I have plenty of energy. I feel as though I have been set free. My quality of life has improved beyond what I thought was possible through the healing power of food.

Psoriasis can be extremely frustrating and difficult to treat. However, there is always hope for healing. Everyone has different experiences and root causes to address, but this book provides the foundational principles to begin your healing journey. You'll learn all about psoriasis and how to take charge of your condition with lifestyle changes. Take the recipes and diet plans provided here and apply them to your own life to experience tremendous symptom relief—and enjoy some delicious food along the way!

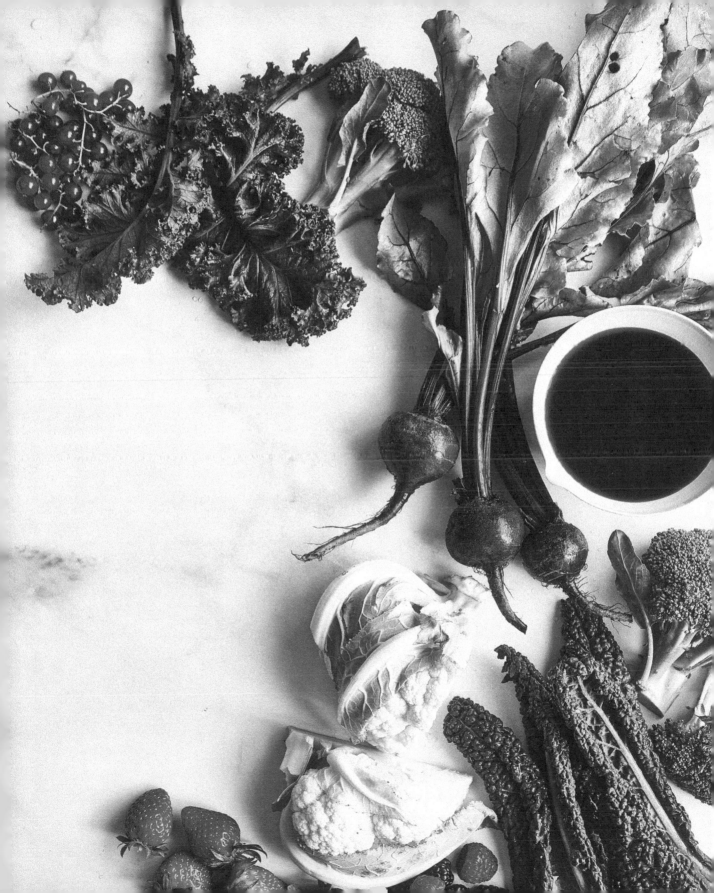

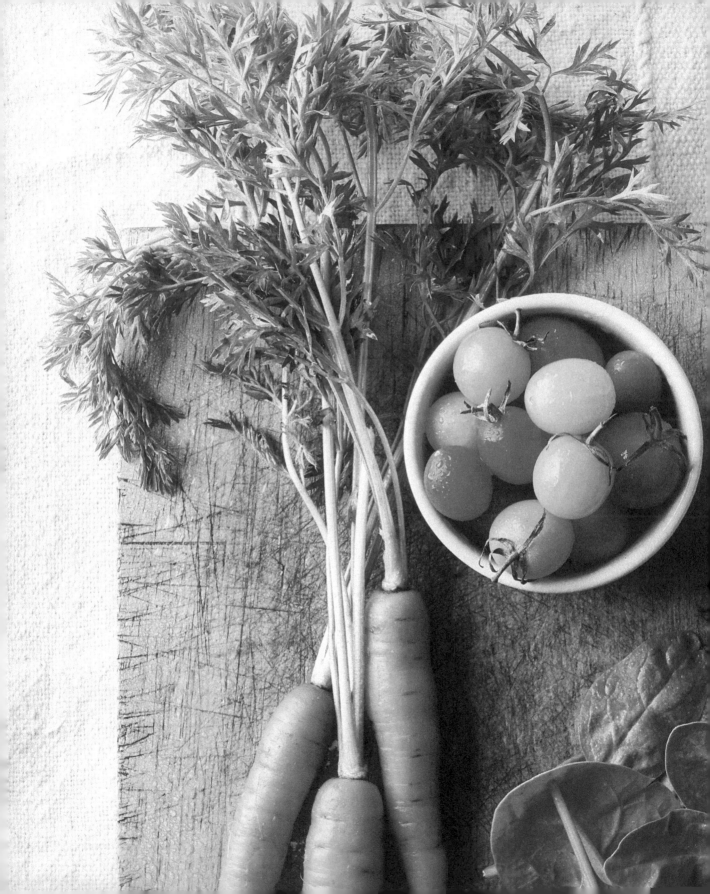

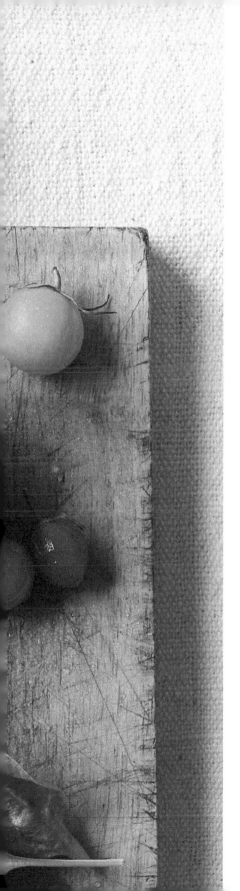

PART ONE
PSORIASIS RELIEF THROUGH DIET

Traditional treatment for psoriasis includes symptom management with tools such as light therapy and medications, but nutrition-related strategies are also becoming an important part of psoriasis treatment protocols.

The standard American diet, which is high in processed and refined foods, additives, dairy, gluten, inflammatory fats, and sugar, has been shown to contribute to the development of diseases like psoriasis. A whole foods, gluten- and dairy-free, plant-centered diet—one that's high in anti-inflammatory compounds and fiber and contains moderate amounts of healthy fat—can lead to dramatic symptom improvement and, possibly, even reverse the disease.

The first two chapters of this book teach you all about the causes, symptoms, and triggers of psoriasis and how diet affects psoriasis symptoms. Chapter 3 presents the meal plans that show you how to incorporate nourishing foods into your diet so you can begin to heal your body from the inside out.

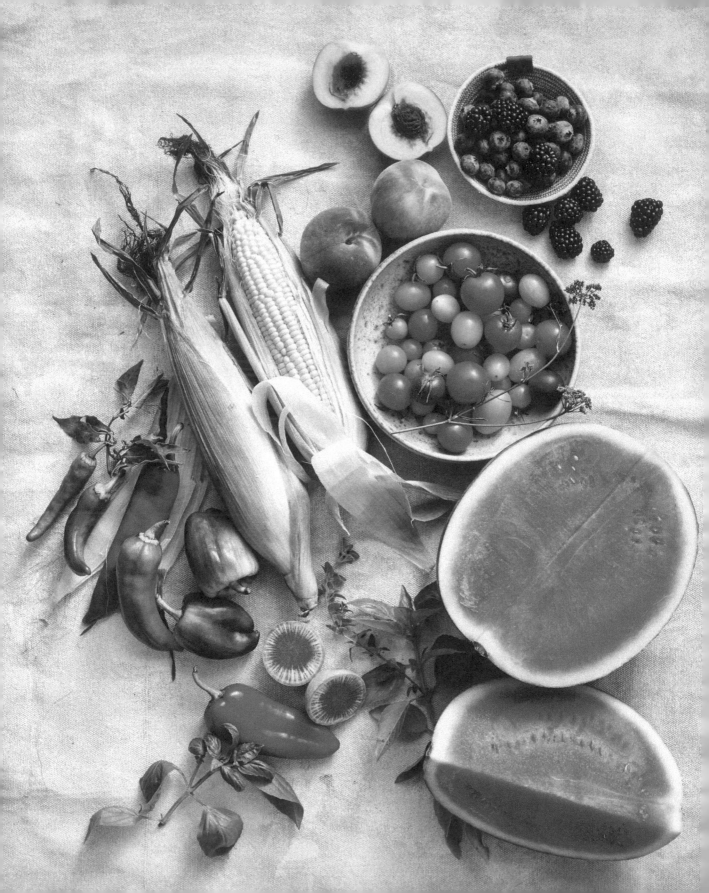

1
ALL ABOUT PSORIASIS

Before you can relieve and reverse the symptoms of psoriasis with nutrition, it's important to understand how this disease develops, the different types of psoriasis, and the variety of symptoms that present.

What Is Psoriasis?

Psoriasis is a chronic inflammatory autoimmune skin disease that affects seven million Americans. There is a strong genetic component to the disease, but anyone can develop psoriasis at any time. Most psoriasis sufferers experience their first symptoms in their mid-teens to early 20s. However, as reported in the journal *Pediatric Drugs*, up to one-third of psoriasis cases now begin in childhood. In fact, childhood psoriasis cases have more than doubled over the past 50 years.

Psoriasis is a noncontagious disease in which skin cells grow at a more rapid pace than normal with altered cell differentiation. Those excess skin cells cover inflammatory substances in the skin, causing the psoriatic lesions. There are several types of psoriasis, including psoriasis vulgaris (plaque psoriasis), guttate, inverse, nail, and pustular. Rarely, erythrodermic psoriasis can occur, which is characterized by 90 percent of the body's total surface area becoming inflamed with psoriatic lesions and requiring emergency treatment.

As reported in the *International Journal of Molecular Sciences*, psoriasis vulgaris (plaque psoriasis) is the most common type of psoriasis and is responsible for 90 percent of all psoriasis cases. People with plaque psoriasis experience red, inflamed areas of skin with silvery, flaky scales commonly presenting on the arms, legs, scalp, and torso. Psoriatic lesions, no matter the type or location, are often itchy and tender and can often bleed. The more they are scratched, the more inflamed they become.

Although the skin symptoms can be extremely painful and frustrating, psoriasis is not limited to its effects on the skin. People with psoriasis are at greater risk for developing psoriatic arthritis, a degenerative joint condition due to the disease's hallmark systemic inflammation. They also face an increased risk of chronic diseases such as metabolic syndrome, cardiovascular disease, depression, inflammatory bowel disease, high blood pressure, fatty liver disease, and type 2 diabetes. In children, psoriasis is associated with higher rates of mental health disorders.

Psoriasis is a chronic relapsing and remitting disease with no known cure. Symptoms typically occur in a cycle, often improving and then getting worse. Although there are a variety of ways to improve psoriasis symptoms, such as with topical creams, vitamin D, light therapy, and medications, nutrition therapy offers relief with the potential to heal the body from the inside out. This book focuses on making dietary changes to start this healing process. To maximize results, it's important to understand the triggers and root causes of psoriasis.

WHEN TO SEE A DOCTOR

Although it's tempting to diagnose yourself with psoriasis, it's always important to speak with a doctor or appropriate specialist if you suspect you have psoriasis. The symptoms of psoriasis may seem recognizable, but there could be other causes for your skin lesions.

In addition, learning the type of psoriasis you have may be important for treatment. The information in this book is appropriate for most forms of psoriasis, but there may be other factors that need to be addressed based on your specific type.

If you have had psoriasis for several years, it's still important to maintain contact with your health care provider—especially if your condition worsens, the lesions spread to new areas or affect a larger percentage of your body, or if you begin to experience joint pain and swelling. If your current treatment plan is no longer effective or if you begin to experience any other physical or mental health symptoms, it's important to seek medical attention.

The meal plans and recipes included in this book are aimed at improving psoriasis symptoms and metabolic health, but remember, everyone is unique and will experience dietary changes differently. It is normal to experience a few days of negative symptoms when starting this type of meal plan. If those symptoms don't improve after the first week or after you've completed the four-week meal plan, follow up with your physician.

Psoriasis Causes and Triggers

Although psoriasis is known to be an immune mediated disease, its exact cause is not known. It does have a strong genetic component, with primary and secondary family members of those with psoriasis being at greater risk for the disease. In addition, identical twins are two to three times more likely to develop psoriasis when compared to fraternal twins.

Psoriasis is characterized by autoimmune and autoinflammatory processes that perpetuate one another. Like other autoimmune and chronic inflammatory diseases, psoriasis requires three factors to develop: a genetic predisposition, an environmental trigger, and increased intestinal permeability. Simply having a genetic predisposition does not mean you will develop psoriasis. In fact, only 10 percent of people with a genetic predisposition ever develop the disease.

Here are some common psoriasis triggers:

- Air pollution, which can increase oxidative stress

- Chronic unmanaged stress, which can significantly affect immune system function

- Excessive alcohol consumption

- Injury to an unaffected area of skin (in patients with psoriasis), causing new lesions to develop

- Prolonged or unprotected sun exposure, which increases oxidative stress

- Smoking and second hand smoke exposure

Some medications can exacerbate preexisting lesions, induce new lesions, or trigger psoriasis in those with or without a family history. The most common medicines, as reported in the *International Journal of Molecular Sciences*, include angiotensin-converting enzyme inhibitors, anti-malarial drugs, beta blockers, fibrates, interferons, lithium, nonsteroidal anti-inflammatory drugs, terbinafine, and tetracycline. Stopping steroid medications abruptly may also be a trigger.

Certain infections, such as streptococcal (strep throat) and staphylococcus (staph) skin infections, can also trigger symptoms of psoriasis. Inflammatory conditions, such as obesity and increased intestinal permeability, also play a role in the disease.

INCREASED INTESTINAL PERMEABILITY

Increased intestinal permeability, or leaky gut, is not classified as a disease itself, but rather is an indication of the inflammation and dysbiosis that underlie many chronic disease conditions, including psoriasis. Dysbiosis is any imbalance or change in the gut microbiome that leads to the symptoms of disease.

Your small intestine is tasked with filtering what should be absorbed into the body (such as properly digested nutrients) and what should exit the body (harmful microbes, undigested food particles, and chemicals). The small intestine lining is held together by tight junctions, which can be affected by the protein zonulin.

With chronic inflammatory diseases such as psoriasis, zonulin is inappropriately released and the small intestinal cell layer becomes more permeable to large food particles, bacteria, and chemicals that should be exiting the body. When increased intestinal permeability is present, these toxins can induce inflammation in the gut, which further increases intestinal permeability. Once these substances cross the protective gut barrier, the body mounts a full defense to rid itself of these invaders, which fuels inflammation and contributes to the development of chronic inflammatory disease symptoms.

There are many potential triggers for the development or exacerbation of psoriasis, and it's important to identify your specific triggers. Although you can't eliminate the genetic predisposition, you can definitely work toward removing known disease triggers and improving your intestinal health. A comprehensive plan for healing should consider how your psoriasis developed and what triggers your symptoms, then implement strategies to begin reversing that process.

Psoriasis Symptoms

Typically, skin cells are replaced every 28 to 30 days, but in people with psoriasis, this process is expedited and occurs every 3 to 5 days. As a result of this rapid cell regeneration, old, dead skin cells are pushed to the outer skin layer, causing the classic silvery, scaly appearance of the affected skin. Underlying this rapid skin cell turnover is inflammation, creating the reddened, raised lesions. While this inflammation and rapid cell turnover is common in all forms of psoriasis, symptoms may be different based on the specific type.

Erythrodermic psoriasis is rare, but it can develop suddenly and, generally, involves lesions covering 90 percent of the body's total surface area.

Guttate psoriasis causes small pink areas with more delicate scales.

Inverse psoriasis involves lesions that are mostly red and swollen, but do not often have the classic silvery scales. These lesions occur in areas of skin folds, like the underarms, under the breasts, and in the genital area.

Nail psoriasis is characterized by pitting and separation of the nail from the nail bed, scaling under the nail, and nail discoloration.

Plaque psoriasis manifests as well-defined swollen red areas typically found on the torso, scalp, knees, elbows, and buttocks. The lesions are generally symmetrical throughout the body and can occur on the palms of the hands, soles of the feet, and over joints, which can be disabling.

Pustular psoriasis involves an increase in neutrophils in the outer skin layer, which can cause pustules to form on the palms of the hands or soles of the feet.

Psoriatic lesions can occur on a small portion of the skin, such as in my case. Or, the lesions can cover many areas of the body. The most common areas include the elbows, face, knees, legs, lower back, and scalp. Lesions are cyclical in nature and can be present for long periods of time before improving and/or disappearing.

SIMPLE STEPS FOR PSORIASIS RELIEF

There is no one food or medication that will cure psoriasis, and it sometimes takes trial and error to find what works to ease your symptoms. While you are working toward healing your body from the inside out, here are some tips to relieve your symptoms along the way.

Add tea tree essential oil to your shampoo: **Anecdotally, this helps reduce the itch from scalp psoriasis.**

Apply cold compresses to reduce inflammation: **Do not apply ice directly to skin, as this can damage the skin, making you more at risk of developing psoriatic lesions. It's best to use a soft, thin towel as a barrier between the ice and the skin.**

Avoid skin injuries: **People with psoriasis are at greater risk of developing lesions when the skin is damaged by a cut or bruise.**

Get out in the sun, but avoid sunburns: **Sun exposure is important to maintain adequate vitamin D levels and has also been shown to improve psoriasis plaques. However, people with psoriasis should avoid extended periods of unprotected time in the sun and avoid sunburns.**

Moisturize: **Use nontoxic skin products to moisturize your skin multiple times throughout the day. Read the labels and avoid products with alcohol, fragrance, parabens, and phthalates.**

Try hemp seed oil: **When applied topically to the skin, hemp seed oil can reduce dryness.**

Try meditation or yoga: **Developing a steady practice can help reduce stress hormone levels in the body and, in turn, decrease inflammation. Check out free online resources tailored for beginners.**

Treating Psoriasis with Food

Many treatment options exist for psoriasis, including ultraviolet light therapy, vitamin D topical cream, and topical and systemic steroids. There are also disease-modifying anti-rheumatic drugs (DMARDs) and injectable biologic medications available for psoriasis sufferers. I had some improvement with topical creams, and my sister, who also suffered from psoriasis, felt light therapy and vitamin D cream were helpful, but neither of us experienced dramatic improvement and reversal of our symptoms until we changed our diet and lifestyle.

Nutrition therapy is an inexpensive, safe treatment option that teaches you how food affects your symptoms. As you learn more about your body's needs, you can personalize your approach and experience long-term symptom relief. People with psoriasis are at increased risk for other autoimmune and chronic inflammatory conditions, which means that learning how to prepare and consume wholesome meals can also improve your overall health.

With all autoimmune diseases, including psoriasis, the body's immune system can no longer distinguish friend from foe. Instead of attacking viruses, bacteria, and parasites that could cause harm to the body, the immune system begins to attack its own healthy tissues and organs, leading to a variety of symptoms and serious consequences. In the case of psoriasis, this leads to more rapid skin cell regeneration and manifests in red, inflamed, scaly plaques, but it can also result in painful, swollen joints, as is the case with psoriatic arthritis.

Targeting the immune system begins with the gut. The majority of the immune system resides in the gastrointestinal tract. When the gut microbiome is out of balance, the immune system is affected. As reported in the *British Medical Journal,* the gut microbiome of people with autoimmune diseases like psoriasis is out of balance when compared to healthy people. This imbalance is partially responsible for the development of increased intestinal permeability and psoriasis symptoms.

The gut microbiome is now known to be one of the most important drivers of health. Many factors can affect your gut microbiome, including age, medications, method of birth, stress, and/or whether you were breast- or bottle-fed as a child. However, your diet has the most important impact on the composition of your gut microbes.

Because people with psoriasis already experience inflammation, it makes sense to avoid foods known to be inflammatory and to eat more foods that fight inflammation. In the next chapter, we'll not only learn which foods to enjoy and avoid, but also how to incorporate inflammation-fighting nutrients into your diet to target your psoriasis symptoms.

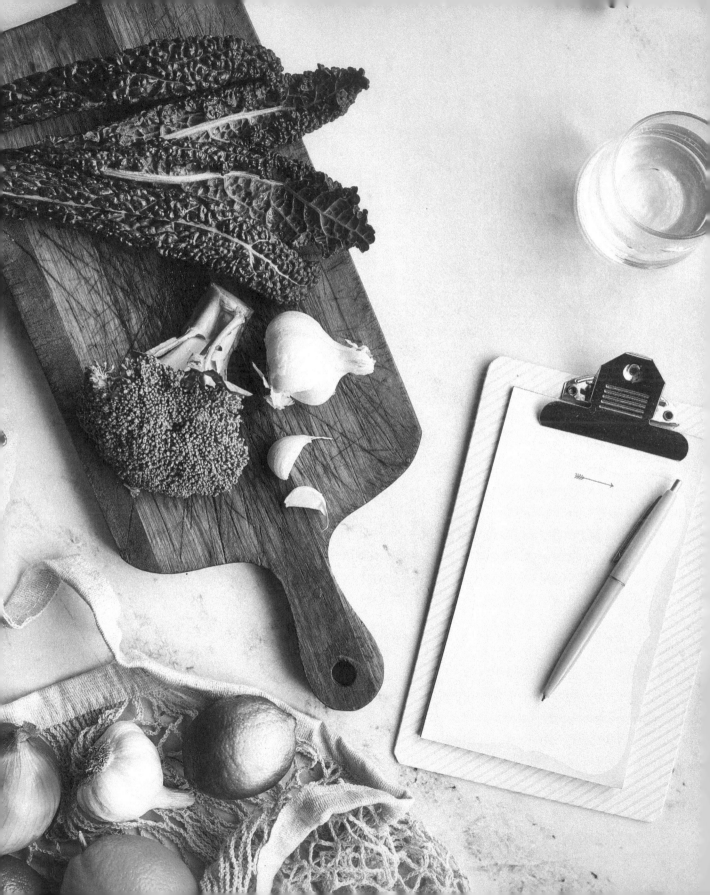

2

THE PSORIASIS-DIET CONNECTION

Healing your body from the inside out starts with the psoriasis meal plan. In this chapter, you'll learn the principles of the psoriasis diet and how food can affect your psoriasis symptoms. By the end of this chapter, you'll know which foods to stock in your kitchen and which to toss out.

Principles of the Psoriasis Diet

If making diet-related changes feels challenging, remember that food can make a big difference for psoriasis. A meal plan based on anti-inflammatory foods and low in inflammation-causing foods can positively and powerfully affect your psoriasis symptoms, prevent flare-ups, and even help reverse the underlying disease.

Like other anti-inflammatory dietary approaches to healing, the psoriasis meal plan in this book is based on the Mediterranean diet, which has been researched extensively and is known to be effective in the treatment and prevention of many chronic diseases. For psoriasis, the Mediterranean diet has been shown to decrease psoriasis severity and even prevent the disease.

The traditional Mediterranean diet is plant-based and high in healthy mono-unsaturated fats, fish, fruits, legumes, nuts, vegetables, and whole grains while also being low in dairy products, eggs, red meat, and alcohol. The meal plan and recipes you'll find in this book take it a step further: eliminating all alcohol, dairy, eggs, and gluten, which can all increase inflammation and negatively impact the gut microbiome for people with autoimmune diseases. Nightshades (a group of vegetables that includes bell peppers, eggplant, tomatoes, and white potatoes) are also limited. Although eggs and nightshades can be part of a healthy diet for most people, they can cause inflammation in some people with autoimmune disease.

In addition to increasing the amount of anti-inflammatory foods in your diet, the psoriasis meal plan can also help you identify foods that trigger your symptoms or flare-ups by having you remove inflammatory foods for a period of time. You may be able to reintroduce some of the eliminated foods, but the process aims to provide you with a better understanding of foods you need to avoid completely.

Under the psoriasis meal plan, I recommend eating three meals per day with minimal to no refined carbohydrates, which will help stabilize blood sugar levels, decrease the risk of metabolic syndrome and type 2 diabetes, and improve your energy level. Avoid eating within three hours of bedtime for more restful sleep.

Foods that Fight Inflammation

No single food is an inflammation cure-all, but you can use diet to create an environment for fighting out-of-control inflammation, as seen in psoriasis. This psoriasis meal plan focuses on anti-inflammatory foods rich in monounsaturated fats, dietary fiber, polyphenols, and antioxidants.

Beans

Beans are an inexpensive source of plant-based protein and are packed with antioxidants, fiber, minerals, and anti-inflammatory benefits. Some people with autoimmune disease avoid beans due to their lectin content, which can disrupt the gastrointestinal lining and fuel inflammation. Soaking beans and cooking them thoroughly deactivates the lectin. Those new to beans in their diet may experience gas but, ultimately, the psoriasis meal plan reduces gas. Dried beans cooked from scratch are best, but canned beans are convenient and already low in lectin.

Fruits and Vegetables

Fruits and vegetables are important sources of antioxidants, dietary fiber, minerals, and vitamins. Fiber is powerful fuel for gut bacteria and promotes the healthy elimination of toxins from the body. A healthy gut microbiome is important for preventing increased intestinal permeability, which can fuel the inflammatory process. To fight inflammation, eat at least nine servings of fruits and vegetables daily, focusing on variety and vegetables. For reference, one serving equals ½ cup of cooked vegetables or 1 cup of raw vegetables.

Gluten-Free Grains

The psoriasis meal plan is lower in grains, but gluten-free whole grains are a great source of fiber, minerals, phytonutrients, and vitamins. Gluten-free grains help keep blood sugar levels stable and fight inflammation, and their fiber content provides gut microbiome fuel. When these grains are cooked and cooled, they offer resistant starch to fuel the gut microbiome. Some good examples include amaranth, brown rice, buckwheat, gluten-free oats, millet, quinoa, sorghum, and teff.

Herbs and Spices

Herbs and spices boost flavor and magnify the antioxidant and anti-inflammatory effects of foods. Black pepper, cinnamon, cloves, ginger, sage, and turmeric offer anti-inflammatory properties. Cinnamon and coriander lower blood sugar, and garlic and ginger improve arthritis symptoms. Cumin and rosemary improve immune system function. Basil, cloves, oregano, sage, and thyme provide antioxidant benefits. Use fresh or dried herbs, which should be stored in a cool, dry place and tossed after one year. To substitute dried herbs for fresh, substitute 1 teaspoon dried for every 1 tablespoon of fresh.

Nuts and Seeds

Nuts can lower blood sugar levels, maintain healthy cholesterol levels, and decrease inflammation. Nuts and seeds are high in monounsaturated, polyunsaturated, and saturated fats—vital for healthy metabolism, brain function, and satiety. Nuts also contain fiber and act as prebiotics for the gut bacteria. Nuts and seeds contain important micronutrients (magnesium and selenium) and are sources of antioxidants. Try almonds, Brazil nuts, cashews, chia seeds, flaxseed, hemp seeds, hazelnuts, macadamia nuts, pecans, pistachios, pumpkin seeds, sesame seeds, and walnuts.

Olive Oil

Extra-virgin olive oil (EVOO) is a Mediterranean diet staple. This mostly monounsaturated fat has anti-inflammatory, antioxidant, and immune-modulating properties—important in controlling blood pressure, insulin levels, and weight. These properties assist in the prevention and treatment of cancer, metabolic and vascular diseases, and inflammatory autoimmune conditions. This healthy fat also contains polyphenolic compounds. Don't use extra-virgin olive oil for high-heat cooking, though, as the healthy fats become unstable at temperatures above 350°F. Instead, drizzle the oil on foods after cooking or use it for salad dressings.

Omega-3 Fatty Acids

Omega-3 fats are powerful for the prevention and treatment of inflammatory conditions such as psoriasis. The two most beneficial omega-3 fats are eicosapentaenoic acid (EPA) and docosahexaenoic acid (DHA), found in fatty fish such as wild-caught salmon, sardines, and tuna, as well as grass-fed beef and pasture-raised eggs. The body cannot make omega-3 fatty acids, so they must be obtained from food. Consume fatty fish at least twice per week. If you don't like fish, ask your health care provider about taking nutritional supplements.

THE POWER OF GREEN TEA

Green tea, a popular beverage in many parts of the world, has been consumed for centuries. This tea is inexpensive and simple to make at home and available in many cafes and restaurants.

Research has shown that green tea has a number of health-promoting benefits. Green tea has been found to inhibit the growth of cancer cells and may play an important role in the prevention of breast, pancreatic, prostate, skin, and stomach cancers, according to the *International Journal of Molecular Sciences*. Green tea has also been shown to have powerful benefits when it comes to diabetes and neurodegenerative and cardiovascular diseases.

Drinking unsweetened green tea daily can be another tool in your toolbox against psoriasis flares, as the polyphenol content of green tea, specifically catechins, provides anti-inflammatory and antioxidant effects. Although green tea powders and supplements are available, it's important to speak with your provider before adding these types of products to your diet.

Inflammatory Foods

Food can be a powerful tool in the prevention and treatment of inflammatory conditions. But food also has the ability to fuel the inflammatory process, creating or worsening diseases such as psoriasis. The psoriasis meal plan restricts or even eliminates foods common in the typical American diet due to their potentially inflammatory effects, but it also recommends delicious alternatives.

Corn, Grain-Fed Meats, and Pork

Although corn is a whole grain, the majority of corn available in the United States is genetically modified (GMO) and highly processed, which may increase inflammation. The psoriasis meal plan does not include corn, but good quality organic, non-GMO corn may be included if you do not have an allergy or sensitivity. Factory-farmed pork and grain-fed meats can also be inflammatory for some people, so the psoriasis meal plan does not include either of those foods.

Dairy

Dairy products are beloved by many, but they can be problematic. Lactose intolerance is common, but in sensitive individuals, dairy can also potentially increase inflammation. I encourage the elimination of most conventional dairy products. There are no dairy products included in the psoriasis meal plan here, but if you decide to continue to consume dairy, look for goat's or sheep's milk, which are usually better tolerated than cow's milk. When possible, choose grass-fed butter, kefir, and yogurt.

Gluten

Gluten is the protein found in barley, rye, and wheat. In grain-based America, gluten is a staple, but it can drive the inflammatory process. For people with celiac disease, gluten must be eliminated. Even in those without a celiac diagnosis, gluten-containing foods can increase intestinal permeability and negative symptoms. The psoriasis meal plan does not include any gluten-containing grains, but it does include oats. Oats can be contaminated with gluten during processing, so choose certified gluten-free oats.

Nightshades

Nightshade vegetables include bell peppers, eggplant, potatoes, and tomatoes and spices such as cayenne pepper, chili powder, paprika, and red pepper flakes.

Nightshades are packed with nutrients and antioxidants, but they can cause inflammation in some people. Not everyone needs to avoid nightshades, and they are included in a few recipes in this book. If you eat one of these recipes, take note of how you feel. If you see an increase in your psoriasis symptoms, eliminate nightshades for three months and then reintroduce each separately to evaluate how your body responds.

Processed Foods

Although processed foods are convenient, they are also typically full of inflammatory ingredients and gut microbiome disruptors. The psoriasis meal plan uses minimally processed ingredients. Although some prepackaged options may work for you, it's important to read food labels. If you see emulsifiers and gums such as carrageenan and xanthan gum, hydrogenated or partially hydrogenated oils, canola oil, corn oil, safflower oil, soybean oil, sunflower oil, and/or artificial colors or flavors, avoid that food.

Soy

Soy is a plant-based protein that contains valuable minerals, phytonutrients, and vitamins. Soy products in their unprocessed, nongenetically modified form are healthy. However, most soy products are highly processed and contaminated with glyphosate, which can increase inflammation. If you eat soy, look for soy in its whole, unprocessed form (edamame, tofu), and in fermented versions (miso, tempeh). Avoid soybean oil and soy protein isolate. There are no soy-containing foods included in this psoriasis meal plan.

Sugar and Artificial Sweeteners

Sugar is added to enhance flavor—especially to processed foods—at the expense of health. The increase in sugar intake is a culprit in the rise of obesity and chronic inflammatory diseases. The psoriasis meal plan includes some natural sugar (fruit, honey, and pure maple syrup for their antioxidants, minerals, and vitamins), but in limited amounts.

Don't replace sugar with artificial sweeteners (aspartame, saccharin), as research shows these disrupt the gut layer and alter the gut microbiome. As reported in *PLOS ONE*, sucralose, aspartame, and acesulfame potassium increase bacteria associated with obesity. The more natural stevia is one non nutritive option, but it should still be limited.

FERMENTED FOODS AND GUT HEALTH

The gut microbiome is front and center these days—for good reason. A balanced gut microbiome drives good health. When in balance, the microbial communities in the gastrointestinal tract strengthen the intestinal lining and immune system. In people with autoimmune diseases, the gut microbiome is altered, which can fuel the inflammatory process. Diet affects the gut microbiome. Follow the psoriasis meal plan to improve your gut microbial balance and quiet the inflammatory process.

One way to improve the gut's microbial balance is to regularly eat fermented foods. Fermenting—the result of microorganisms converting the carbohydrates in a food to lactic acid—preserves foods and creates beneficial probiotic bacteria. Fermented foods improve digestive function, support a healthy immune system, increase nutrient absorption, and alleviate symptoms of depression and anxiety, as reported in a 2019 review in *Nutrients*. When added to a healthy meal plan, fermented foods can lower blood pressure, blood sugar, and cholesterol levels.

The psoriasis meal plan includes fermented foods such as apple cider vinegar with the mother. Other options include fermented vegetables and pickles, grass-fed yogurt and kefir, kimchi, kombucha, organic non-GMO miso and tempeh, natto, and sauerkraut.

Psoriasis Diet Kitchen Essentials

To successfully implement the psoriasis meal plan, you'll need to use your kitchen. You likely have basic ingredients and kitchen equipment already. Consider investing in items such as storage containers and pantry staples. These will be used frequently and pay for themselves quickly.

Fridge Staples

Store-bought fresh and frozen ingredients are mainstays of the anti-inflammatory recipes included in this book. Choose organic fruits and vegetables when available, look for wild-caught seafood, and opt for organic, pasture-raised poultry.

- Apples
- Arugula
- Asparagus
- Blackberries
- Blueberries
- Carrots
- Cauliflower (fresh and frozen)
- Cherries (frozen)
- Chicken breasts and thighs
- Coconut yogurt
- Coconut milk

- Cod
- Cucumber
- Dandelion greens
- Kale
- Peaches (frozen)
- Pineapple (frozen)
- Red cabbage
- Salmon
- Spinach
- Turkey, ground

Pantry Staples

Many common pantry staples— condiments, dry goods, herbs, oils, and spices —are used in the meal plan recipes for flavor and convenience.

- Almonds, almond butter (no added oil or sugar), and almond flour

- Apple cider vinegar with the mother
- Avocado oil

- Balsamic vinegar
- Black beans (dried or canned)
- Black pepper, freshly ground
- Cashews and cashew butter (no added oil or sugar)
- Chia seeds, hemp seeds, and whole-milled flaxseed
- Chickpeas (dried or canned)
- Coconut flour and coconut oil
- Dijon mustard
- Extra-virgin olive oil
- Gluten-free oats
- Great northern beans (dried or canned)
- Herbs and spices: dried basil, oregano, rosemary, thyme; ground cinnamon, cloves, coriander, cumin, ginger, and turmeric
- Kosher and sea salt
- Pecans and pecan butter (no added oil or sugar)
- Pepitas (pumpkin seeds)
- Quinoa
- Walnuts

Tools and Equipment

All of the psoriasis meal plan recipes require common kitchen equipment and storage containers.

- Blender
- Dutch oven
- Food processor
- Mason jars, small and large
- Measuring cups and spoons
- Mixing bowls, different sizes
- Mixing spoon
- Rubber spatula
- Sheet pan
- Skillet or wok (small, medium, and large)
- Spatula
- Storage containers, different sizes

Making a Psoriasis Diet Work for You

It can be challenging to change what you eat and your daily meal routine. Reversing the inflammatory process of psoriasis requires an anti-inflammatory meal plan. Powering through any negative symptoms that may occur during the first week of the program will allow you to take advantage of all the benefits that healthy, anti-inflammatory foods have to offer. Here are some tips to make your transition more successful.

1. **Eat routine meals.** Eating three meals every day allows you to consume a wide variety of nutrients. Skipping meals can leave you nutrient-depleted and negatively affect blood sugar levels, zapping your energy.

2. **Avoid eating within three hours of bedtime.** When you eat right before bed, your body must switch from relaxation mode to digestion, which requires energy. Allowing the digestion process to complete before bedtime provides a more restful, restorative sleep.

3. **Create a symptom journal.** We are all unique and need a personalized approach to healing. Keeping a symptom journal allows you to link food intake with symptoms. Keeping a journal can also serve as motivation for your healing journey.

4. **Keep your kitchen organized.** It's easier to prepare meals and stay on track in a clean, organized workspace. Clutter can make preparing new foods frustrating.

5. **Consider batch cooking your meals and snacks.** Most of us have hectic schedules, and making meals from scratch on workdays can be difficult. To avoid giving up and ordering out, take a few hours each week to review your meal plan and batch cook for busy days.

6. **Buy canned, frozen, and precut items.** To save time in the kitchen, look for items that can be purchased in canned, frozen, or pre cut forms. Don't skimp on quality, though.

7. **Pack meals and snacks when traveling.** Eating out on the psoriasis meal plan is difficult, especially when traveling. Instead of relying on whatever is available, make your meals and snacks ahead and stock the cooler for travel.

8. **Plan ahead for get-togethers.** When you have a get-together with friends or family, ask about the menu and offer to bring a dish that's appropriate for your psoriasis meal plan.

9. **Stay hydrated.** Oftentimes, we snack thinking we're hungry, but really we're just mildly dehydrated. Keep a container of water close by and drink it often throughout the day. A good rule of thumb is to divide your weight (in pounds) by two. The number you get is how many ounces of water to drink each day.

10. **Give yourself a break.** While following the psoriasis meal plan closely offers the best outcome, be realistic and know that no one is perfect. If you have a bad day, don't be too hard on yourself!

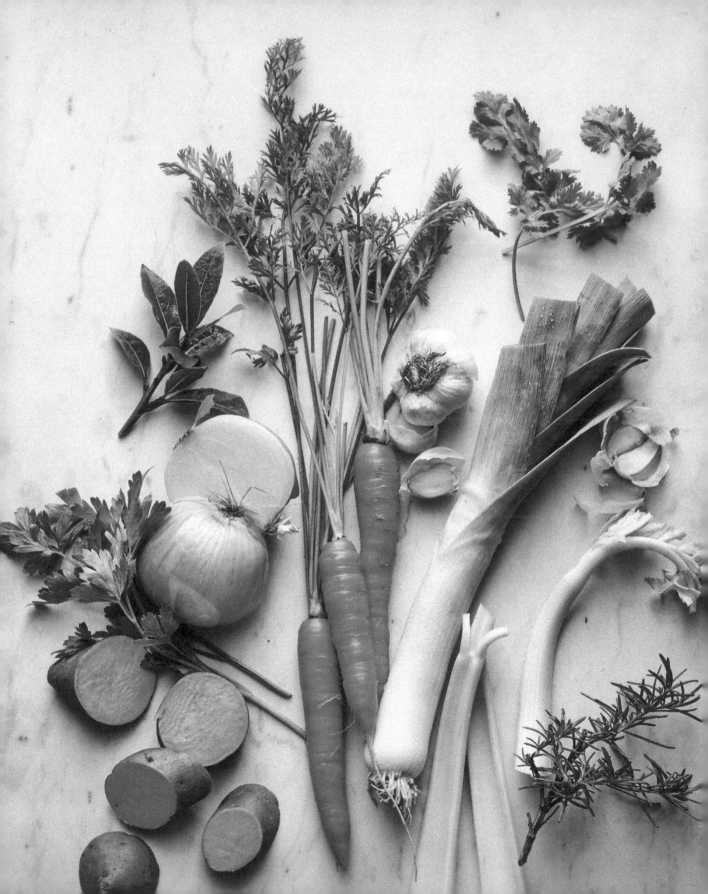

3
THE PSORIASIS DIET PLAN

Changing your diet can feel intimidating. To get you started on your healing journey and make this transition easier, you'll find four psoriasis-friendly meal plans in this chapter. All the information you need is right at your fingertips in an easy-to-use format.

About the Plans

These psoriasis meal plans introduce you to anti-inflammatory recipes that are full of dietary fiber, antioxidants, monounsaturated fats, polyphenols, and other important nutrients your body needs to heal. After starting the meal plans, you may experience relief from your most bothersome psoriasis symptoms.

Each weekly meal plan is designed for one person and includes breakfast, lunch, and dinner. However, the recipes can easily be adjusted for additional servings. There are no snacks in the meal plans, but you can snack on any of the Foods that Fight Inflammation (page 14) or choose from the recipes in chapter 9. Keep snacking to a minimum and avoid eating within three hours of bedtime.

We all have different food preferences, so make substitutions as long as you are choosing wholesome, anti-inflammatory foods. Simply substitute a meal plan recipe with one of the recipes from part 2 of this book.

The meal plans do not include nightshades, which can be inflammatory for some people with psoriasis. There are very few nightshade recipes in part 2, so if you tolerate nightshades, make substitutions where appropriate. If you are unsure whether they are problematic, eliminate them for four weeks. Then, reintroduce them and observe your symptoms. For example, on day one, eat a serving of nightshades twice that day, avoid them on days two and three, then observe for negative symptoms. If you do not notice any change, then it is likely okay to continue eating nightshades. If you do experience a negative symptom, avoid that food for three months before attempting a reintroduction.

By the end of the four-week meal plan, you should have a great foundation for psoriasis-friendly cooking, but the journey doesn't stop there. I encourage you to continue developing your own meal plans based on the recipes included here or modify your own recipes to be anti-inflammatory.

Week 1

During this first week, you may feel sluggish or experience a temporary increase in your symptoms. This is normal and usually lasts only a few days. Instead of giving up, trust the process. Focus on hydration and stress management techniques.

Week 1 of the meal plan increases your intake of green leafy vegetables, lean protein, and dietary fiber and sets the stage for your new anti-inflammatory lifestyle. This is not a calorie-restricted plan, so add any of the nightshade-free recipes from part 2 if you need more food.

Recipes in *italics* indicate leftovers.

	Breakfast	Lunch	Dinner
Mon	Almond Butter and Honey Overnight Oats (page 48)	Turnip and Greens Soup (page 66)	Garlic Chicken and Cauliflower Rice (page 98)
Tue	Cherry-Berry Green Smoothie (page 43)	Mediterranean Tuna Salad (page 74)	*Garlic Chicken and Cauliflower Rice*
Wed	*Almond Butter and Honey Overnight Oats*	*Turnip and Greens Soup*	*Mediterranean Tuna Salad*
Thu	*Cherry-Berry Green Smoothie*	*Mediterranean Tuna Salad*	Mushroom-Zucchini Sauté (page 62)
Fri	*Almond Butter and Honey Overnight Oats*	*Turnip and Greens Soup*	*Mediterranean Tuna Salad*
Sat	Root Vegetable Breakfast Skillet (page 53)	Apple-Curry Turkey Salad (page 92)	*Mushroom-Zucchini Sauté*
Sun	*Root Vegetable Breakfast Skillet*	*Turnip and Greens Soup*	*Apple-Curry Turkey Salad* Garlic Brussels Sprouts (page 129)

Shopping List

This first week you'll pick up staple items to use during the four-week meal plan, so you may spend more money than normal. Check your pantry to see if you have any of the items needed first, then use this list to guide your shopping.

PRODUCE

- ☐ Apple, Gala (1 medium)
- ☐ Arugula (8 cups)
- ☐ Asparagus (6 spears)
- ☐ Avocado, ripe (1)
- ☐ Basil (1 large bunch)
- ☐ Broccoli (1 medium head)
- ☐ Brussels sprouts (1 pound)
- ☐ Carrots (6 medium)
- ☐ Celery stalks (2)
- ☐ Cucumber (1 medium)
- ☐ Garlic (3 heads)
- ☐ Ginger, fresh (1 hand)
- ☐ Lemons (3)
- ☐ Lime (1)
- ☐ Mixed greens (16 cups)
- ☐ Mushrooms, baby bella (1 pound)
- ☐ Onion, red (1 large, 2 medium)
- ☐ Onion, yellow (3 medium)
- ☐ Spinach (6 cups)
- ☐ Sweet potato (2)
- ☐ Swiss chard (1 bunch)
- ☐ Turnips, purple-top (7 medium)
- ☐ Yellow squash (1 medium)
- ☐ Zucchini (2 medium)

REFRIGERATED

- ☐ Nut or seed milk, unsweetened (4 cups)
- ☐ Yogurt, coconut, unsweetened (½ cup)

MEAT AND SEAFOOD

- ☐ Chicken, boneless, skinless breasts (1 pound)
- ☐ Turkey breast, cooked (1 pound)

FROZEN

- ☐ Blueberries (1 cup)
- ☐ Cherries (½ cup)
- ☐ Riced cauliflower (3 cups)

HERBS AND SPICES

- ☐ Bay leaves (2)
- ☐ Black pepper, freshly ground
- ☐ Celery salt

- ☐ Cinnamon, ground
- ☐ Coriander, ground
- ☐ Cumin, ground
- ☐ Dry mustard
- ☐ Garlic powder
- ☐ Ginger, ground
- ☐ Italian seasoning
- ☐ Oregano, dried
- ☐ Sea salt
- ☐ Thyme, dried
- ☐ Turmeric, ground

PANTRY

- ☐ Almond butter
- ☐ Broth, low-sodium vegetable (7¼ cups)
- ☐ Cacao powder
- ☐ Cashew butter
- ☐ Chia seeds (2 tablespoons)
- ☐ Chickpeas (1 [15-ounce] can)
- ☐ Coconut aminos, soy-free (½ cup)
- ☐ Coconut flour (1 tablespoon)
- ☐ Coconut sugar (1 teaspoon)

- ☐ Cranberries, dried (⅓ cup)
- ☐ Flaxseed, whole-milled (¼ cup)
- ☐ Hemp seeds, whole shelled (1 cup)
- ☐ Honey (¼ cup)
- ☐ Lentils, dried green (½ cup)
- ☐ Mustard, Dijon (2 tablespoons)
- ☐ Oats, certified gluten-free, rolled (1¼ cups)
- ☐ Oil, avocado (1 cup)
- ☐ Oil, extra-virgin olive (1½ cups)
- ☐ Olives, green (20)
- ☐ Tuna, water-packed (2 [5-ounce] cans)
- ☐ Vanilla extract
- ☐ Vinegar, apple cider with the mother
- ☐ Vinegar, balsamic
- ☐ Walnuts, chopped (¾ cup)

OTHER

- ☐ Acacia powder (optional)
- ☐ Collagen peptides, vanilla (optional)
- ☐ Vegan protein powder, chocolate

Week 2

Welcome to Week 2. You are likely already experiencing the benefits of this new way of eating. If you haven't noticed positive changes in your symptoms, don't give up. Everyone has a different healing journey. In Week 2, there are more anti-inflammatory spices and vegetables. This week also includes one of my favorite recipes—Carrot Salad with Spicy Greens, topped with Spiced Falafel Balls. This dish bursts with flavor.

	Breakfast	Lunch	Dinner
Mon	Blackberry-Walnut Breakfast Quinoa (page 49)	Apple-Curry Turkey Salad (from Week 1)	Pesto Chicken "Pasta" (page 100) Garlic Brussels Sprouts (from Week 1)
Tue	Root Vegetable Breakfast Skillet (from Week 1)	Pesto Chicken "Pasta" Garlic Brussels Sprouts (from Week 1)	Apple-Curry Turkey Salad (from Week 1) Anti-Inflammatory Cauliflower Soup (page 122)
Wed	Root Vegetable Breakfast Skillet (from Week 1)	Anti-Inflammatory Cauliflower Soup Tuna Lettuce Wraps (page 75)	Pesto Chicken "Pasta" Carrot Salad with Spicy Greens (page 124)
Thu	Blackberry-Walnut Breakfast Quinoa	Carrot Salad with Spicy Greens Pesto Chicken "Pasta"	Anti-Inflammatory Cauliflower Soup Tuna Lettuce Wraps
Fri	Blackberry-Walnut Breakfast Quinoa	Anti-Inflammatory Cauliflower Soup Tuna Lettuce Wraps	Carrot Salad with Spicy Greens Spiced Falafel Balls (page 69)
Sat	Blackberry-Walnut Breakfast Quinoa	Tuna Lettuce Wraps	Carrot Salad with Spicy Greens Spiced Falafel Balls
Sun	Baked Cranberry-Pecan Oatmeal (page 50)	Black Bean Salad with Creamy Avocado Dressing (page 57)	Sheet Pan Mediterranean Chicken (page 104)

Shopping List

You may have some items leftover from Week 1, so be sure to check your stock, especially your pantry items. You may not need to purchase items with an asterisk (*) again for Week 2.

PRODUCE

- ☐ Apple (1 large)
- ☐ Arugula (6 cups)
- ☐ Avocados (2 medium)
- ☐ Blackberries (2 cups)
- ☐ Broccoli (1 large head)
- ☐ Cabbage, red (1 head)
- ☐ Carrots (3 large, 2 medium)
- ☐ Cauliflower (1 small head)
- ☐ Celery (2 stalks)
- ☐ Cucumber (1 small, 1 medium)
- ☐ Garlic (2 heads)
- ☐ Ginger, fresh, grated (1 tablespoon)*
- ☐ Lemons (2)
- ☐ Lettuce, butter (1 large head)
- ☐ Lettuce, red or green leaf (1 head)
- ☐ Limes (2)
- ☐ Mint (1 bunch)
- ☐ Onion, red (1 medium, 1 large)
- ☐ Onion, yellow (1 small)
- ☐ Potatoes, sweet (2 medium)
- ☐ Rutabaga (1 large)
- ☐ Scallions (3 bunches)
- ☐ Spaghetti squash (1 large)
- ☐ Spinach (2 cups)
- ☐ Squash, yellow (1 large)
- ☐ Zucchini (1 large)

REFRIGERATED

- ☐ Nut or seed milk, unsweetened (4 cups)

MEAT AND SEAFOOD

- ☐ Chicken, boneless, skinless breasts (2 pounds)

HERBS AND SPICES

- ☐ Basil, dried
- ☐ Black pepper, freshly ground
- ☐ Cinnamon, ground*
- ☐ Coriander, ground*
- ☐ Cumin, ground*
- ☐ Dill weed, dried
- ☐ Oregano, dried*

□ Parsley, dried

□ Sea salt

□ Turmeric, ground*

PANTRY

□ Black beans (1 [15-ounce] can)

□ Broth, low-sodium vegetable (4 cups)

□ Chickpeas (2 [15-ounce] cans)

□ Coconut oil

□ Coconut sugar (3 tablespoons)^

□ Cranberries, dried (1¼ cups)

□ Flour, gluten-free oat (¼ cup)

□ Hemp seeds, whole shelled (¼ cup)*

□ Honey*

□ Mustard, Dijon*

□ Oats, certified gluten-free, rolled (1½ cups)

□ Oil, avocado (1 cup)*

□ Oil, extra-virgin olive (1½ cups)*

□ Pecans, chopped (¾ cup)

□ Quinoa (1 cup)

□ Tuna, water-packed (2 [5-ounce] cans)

□ Vanilla extract*

□ Vinegar, apple cider vinegar with the mother*

□ Walnuts, chopped (1½ cups)

Week 3

By Week 3, you likely feel more comfortable in the kitchen and have a better understanding of how food might affect your symptoms. Week 3 of the meal plan features delicious Pumpkin-Flax Muffins, which are great served with nut butter. You'll also reap the anti-inflammatory and digestion-promoting benefits of ginger in the scrumptious Pineapple-Ginger Smoothie.

	Breakfast	**Lunch**	**Dinner**
Mon	Baked Cranberry-Pecan Oatmeal (from Week 2)	Sheet Pan Mediterranean Chicken (from Week 2)	Black Bean Salad with Creamy Avocado Dressing (from Week 2)
Tue	Pineapple-Ginger Smoothie (page 46)	Black Bean Salad with Creamy Avocado Dressing (from Week 2)	Sheet Pan Mediterranean Chicken (from Week 2)
Wed	Baked Cranberry-Pecan Oatmeal (from Week 2)	Strawberry and Spinach Salad (page 58)	Sheet Pan Mediterranean Chicken (from Week 2)
Thu	Pineapple-Ginger Smoothie	Black Bean Salad with Creamy Avocado Dressing (from Week 2)	Nut and Oat–Crusted Cod (page 79) Roasted Cauliflower "Steaks" (page 128)
Fri	Baked Cranberry-Pecan Oatmeal (from Week 2)	Strawberry and Spinach Salad Roasted Cauliflower "Steaks"	Nut and Oat–Crusted Cod Simple Roasted Vegetables (page 126)
Sat	Pumpkin-Flax Muffins (page 52) with 1 tablespoon almond butter	Nut and Oat–Crusted Cod Roasted Cauliflower "Steaks"	Crispy Lentil Burgers (page 70) Simple Roasted Vegetables
Sun	Pumpkin-Flax Muffins with 1 tablespoon almond butter	Crispy Lentil Burgers Simple Roasted Vegetables	Nut and Oat–Crusted Cod Roasted Cauliflower "Steaks"

Shopping List

You may have some items leftover from Week 1, so be sure to check your stock, especially your pantry items. You may not need to purchase items with an asterisk (*) again for Week 3.

PRODUCE

- ☐ Avocado (1 large)
- ☐ Banana (1 large)
- ☐ Carrot (1 large)
- ☐ Cauliflower (2 large heads plus 2 cups florets)
- ☐ Celery stalk (1)*
- ☐ Garlic (1 small head)
- ☐ Ginger, fresh, grated (1 teaspoon)*
- ☐ Kohlrabi (1 large, 1 medium)
- ☐ Lemons (3)
- ☐ Mushrooms, baby bella (1 cup chopped, 1 cup sliced)
- ☐ Onion, red (1 small)
- ☐ Pineapple, chunks (1 cup)
- ☐ Radish, daikon (1 medium)
- ☐ Spinach (8 cups)
- ☐ Squash, yellow (1 medium)
- ☐ Strawberries (10 medium)
- ☐ Zucchini (1 medium)

REFRIGERATED

- ☐ Nut or seed milk, unsweetened (2½ cups)

MEAT AND SEAFOOD

- ☐ Cod fillets (4 [6-ounce] fillets)

HERBS AND SPICES

- ☐ Basil, dried*
- ☐ Black pepper, freshly ground
- ☐ Cinnamon, ground*
- ☐ Cumin, ground*
- ☐ Garlic powder*
- ☐ Nutmeg, ground
- ☐ Oregano, dried*
- ☐ Sea salt
- ☐ Thyme, dried*

PANTRY

- ☐ Almond butter
- ☐ Almonds, raw (½ cup)
- ☐ Baking soda
- ☐ Black pepper, freshly ground*

- ☐ Chia seeds (2 tablespoons)*
- ☐ Coconut flour (½ cup)*
- ☐ Flaxseed, whole-milled (7 tablespoons)*
- ☐ Flour, gluten-free oat (½ cup)*
- ☐ Honey*
- ☐ Lentils, green or brown (1 [15-ounce] can)
- ☐ Maple syrup (2 tablespoons)
- ☐ Mustard, Dijon*
- ☐ Oats, certified gluten-free, rolled (1 cup)*
- ☐ Oil, avocado (¾ cup)
- ☐ Oil, coconut (½ cup)

- ☐ Oil, extra-virgin olive (½ cup)
- ☐ Pecans, raw (½ cup)
- ☐ Pepitas (sunflower seeds), raw (½ cup)
- ☐ Pumpkin, pure (1 [15-ounce] can)
- ☐ Sea salt*
- ☐ Vanilla extract*
- ☐ Walnuts, raw, chopped (1 cup)

OTHER

- ☐ Collagen peptides, vanilla (optional)*
- ☐ Vegan protein powder, vanilla (2 scoops)*

Week 4

Congratulations on making it to Week 4! You should be proud of yourself. Even if you've encountered some hiccups along the way, remember: This journey is a marathon, not a sprint. By now you will have discovered some delicious alternatives to your favorite foods. In Week 4, we're focusing on plant-based meals with limited animal products to maximize phytonutrient intake, further decrease inflammation, and promote optimal digestion.

	Breakfast	Lunch	Dinner
Mon	*Pumpkin-Flax Muffins (from Week 3)* with 1 tablespoon almond butter	Easy Vegan Hummus Bowl (page 61)	Leek and Kohlrabi Stir-Fry (page 63)
Tue	Chocolate-Fig Smoothie (page 44)	*Crispy Lentil Burgers (from Week 3) Simple Roasted Vegetables (from Week 3)*	*Easy Vegan Hummus Bowl*
Wed	*Pumpkin-Flax Muffins (from Week 3)* with 1 tablespoon almond butter	*Easy Vegan Hummus Bowl*	*Leek and Kohlrabi Stir-Fry*
Thu	*Chocolate-Fig Smoothie*	*Leek and Kohlrabi Stir-Fry*	Sheet Pan Almond-Butter Salmon and Broccoli (page 87)
Fri	*Pumpkin-Flax Muffins (from Week 3)* with 1 tablespoon almond butter	*Sheet Pan Almond-Butter Salmon and Broccoli*	Tangy Chicken with Quinoa (page 97)
Sat	*Pumpkin-Flax Muffins (from Week 3)* with 1 tablespoon almond butter	*Leek and Kohlrabi Stir-Fry*	*Sheet Pan Almond-Butter Salmon and Broccoli*
Sun	Purple Cruciferous Berry Smoothie (page 47)	*Sheet Pan Almond-Butter Salmon and Broccoli*	*Tangy Chicken with Quinoa*

Shopping List

You may have some items leftover from Week 1, so be sure to check your stock, especially your pantry items. You may not need to purchase items with an asterisk (*) again for Week 4.

PRODUCE

- ☐ Avocados (2 medium)
- ☐ Banana (1 medium)
- ☐ Blueberries (1 cup)
- ☐ Broccoli (1 large head)
- ☐ Cabbage, red (1 small)
- ☐ Carrot (1 medium)
- ☐ Cucumber (1 mini)
- ☐ Fig (1; or 2 dried)
- ☐ Garlic (5 cloves)
- ☐ Greens, mixed (8 cups)
- ☐ Kale, curly, chopped (2 cups)
- ☐ Kohlrabi (2 medium)
- ☐ Leeks (4 medium)
- ☐ Lemon (1)
- ☐ Lime (1)
- ☐ Scallions (4)
- ☐ Spinach (9 cups)
- ☐ Sweet potato (1 medium)
- ☐ Swiss chard, chopped (6 cups)

REFRIGERATED

- ☐ Nut or seed milk, unsweetened (5 cups)

MEAT AND SEAFOOD

- ☐ Salmon (4 [6-ounce] fillets)

FROZEN

- ☐ Blueberries (2 cups)

HERBS AND SPICES

- ☐ Basil, dried*
- ☐ Black pepper, freshly ground
- ☐ Cinnamon, ground*
- ☐ Coriander, dried*
- ☐ Cumin, ground*
- ☐ Dill weed, dried*
- ☐ Garlic powder*
- ☐ Ginger, ground*
- ☐ Italian seasoning*
- ☐ Sea salt

PANTRY

- ☐ Almond butter
- ☐ Beans, cannellini (1 [15-ounce] can)

- ☐ Cacao powder (1 tablespoon)*
- ☐ Cashews, dry-roasted (1 cup)
- ☐ Chia seeds (2 tablespoons)*
- ☐ Chicken breast, shredded (2 [12.5-ounce] cans)
- ☐ Chickpeas (3 [15-ounce] cans)
- ☐ Coconut aminos, soy-free (¼ cup)*
- ☐ Flaxseed, whole-milled (2 tablespoons)*
- ☐ Hemp seeds, whole shelled (¼ cup)
- ☐ Honey*
- ☐ Mustard, Dijon*
- ☐ Oil, avocado (2 tablespoons)*
- ☐ Oil, extra-virgin olive (1½ cups)
- ☐ Pepitas, raw (½ cup)
- ☐ Quinoa, red (1 cup)
- ☐ Quinoa, white (1 cup; or 2 cups cooked)
- ☐ Vinegar, apple cider with the mother (½ cup)*
- ☐ Vinegar, balsamic (6 tablespoons)*

OTHER

- ☐ Acacia powder (optional)*
- ☐ Collagen peptides, vanilla (optional)*
- ☐ Vegan protein powder, chocolate*
- ☐ Vegan protein powder, vanilla*

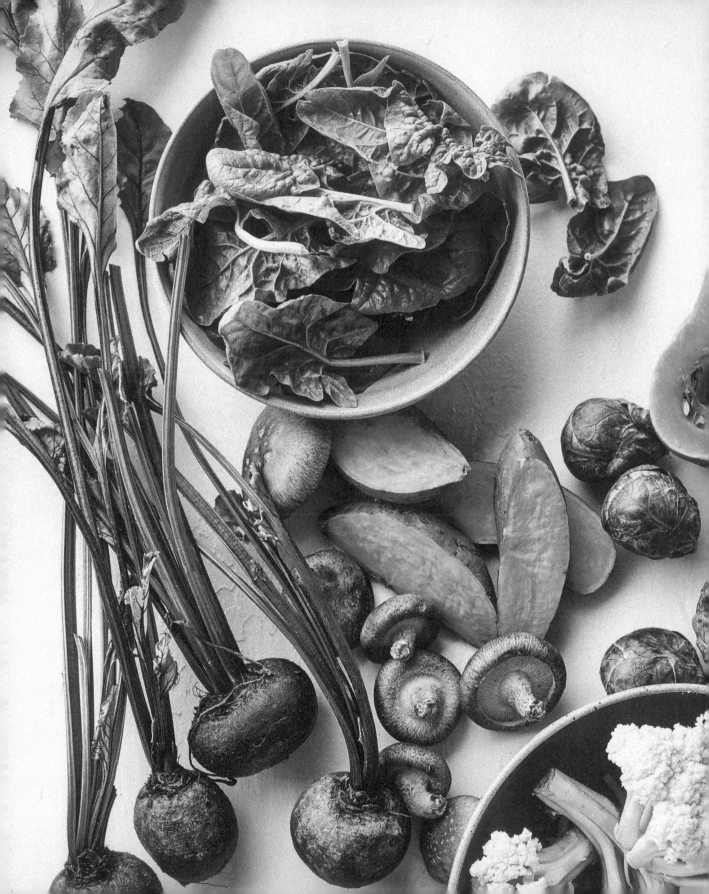

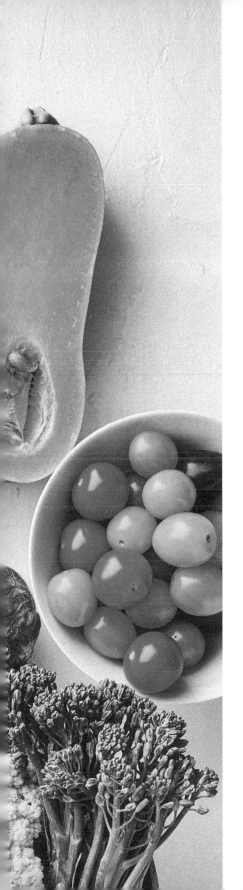

PART TWO
RECIPES FOR PSORIASIS RELIEF

In the following chapters, you'll find 75 anti-inflammatory, psoriasis-friendly recipes designed to help you continue your healing journey. During your four-week meal plan, you can substitute any of the nightshade-free options for any recipe in the meal plan. Once you've completed the four weeks of meal plans, you can begin testing recipes that include nightshades. You'll find labels for each recipe: dairy-free, gluten-free, nightshade-free, vegan, or vegetarian. Aside from being delicious, the recipes are easy-to-make and use simple, wholesome, easy-to-find ingredients that target inflammation and soothe your psoriasis symptoms.

Each recipe includes information about the nutrients found in that dish and how they may be important for psoriasis sufferers. To make the transition to anti-inflammatory cooking even easier, you'll find helpful information about cooking with certain ingredients, making substitutions, varying the recipe, batch cooking, and easier preparation techniques. You'll also find nutritional information for each recipe.

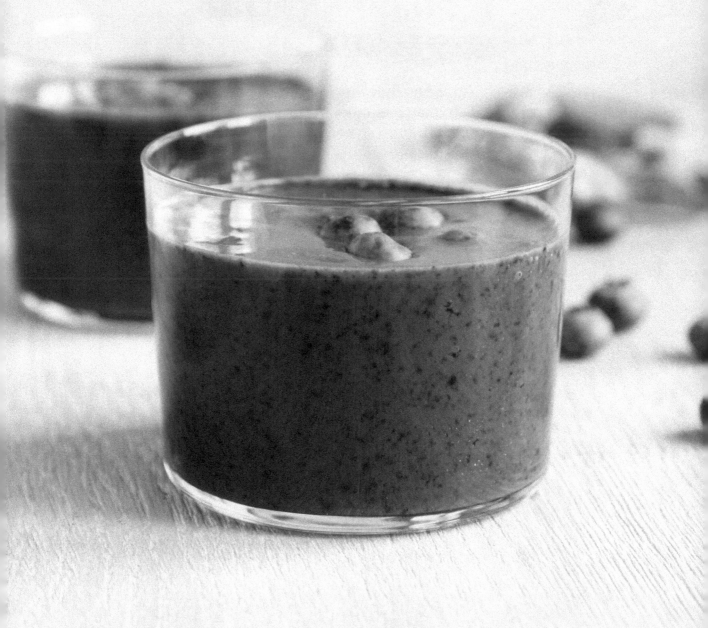

Cherry-Berry Green Smoothie, page 43

4

BREAKFASTS AND SMOOTHIES

Mintalicious Green Smoothie

DAIRY-FREE, GLUTEN-FREE, NIGHTSHADE-FREE

SERVES 2 PREP TIME: 10 minutes

Adding fresh herbs, like mint, to your daily routine is a great way to increase your intake of antioxidants and aid healthy digestion. The optional collagen peptides in this smoothie offer another way to boost gut health. Collagen is the most abundant protein in the body, but our ability to produce collagen decreases as we age. Collagen is not only important for healthy bones, joints, and skin, but it may also help heal the gut lining and prevent increased intestinal permeability.

2½ cups unsweetened nut or seed milk (almond, coconut, flax, or hemp seed)

1 tablespoon cacao powder

½ teaspoon vanilla extract

1 scoop vanilla collagen peptides (optional)

1 scoop vegan vanilla protein powder

2 small frozen bananas

2 cups fresh spinach

3 fresh mint leaves

In a blender, combine the nut milk, cacao powder, vanilla, collagen peptides (if using), protein powder, bananas, spinach, and mint. Blend on high speed for 1 minute, until smooth.

> **Ingredient tip:** Collagen peptides and vegan protein powder are found in most grocery stores. You can also order organic varieties online. To make any of the smoothie recipes vegan, omit the collagen peptides.

Per Serving: Calories: 222; Total Fat: 6g; Saturated Fat: <1g; Cholesterol: 0mg; Carbohydrates: 37g; Fiber: 7g; Protein: 14g

Cherry-Berry Green Smoothie

DAIRY-FREE, GLUTEN-FREE, NIGHTSHADE-FREE
SERVES 2 PREP TIME: 10 minutes

This mouthwatering smoothie is loaded with polyphenols, which are important for lowering inflammation. Cherries provide flavor, vitamin C to support a healthy immune system, and fiber to fuel the gut microbiome. Cherries also help post-exercise recovery, making this a good after-exercise snack. The optional acacia powder is a great option for enhancing the gut microbiome.

2½ cups unsweetened nut or seed milk (almond, coconut, flax, or hemp seed)

2 cups fresh spinach

1 cup frozen blueberries

½ cup frozen cherries

2 tablespoons cashew butter or Pumpkin Seed Butter (page 127)

1 scoop vanilla collagen peptides (optional)

1 scoop vegan chocolate protein powder

2 tablespoons chia seeds

1 teaspoon ground cinnamon

2 teaspoons acacia powder (optional)

1 tablespoon cacao powder

In a blender, combine the nut milk, spinach, blueberries, cherries, cashew butter, collagen peptides (if using), protein powder, chia seeds, cinnamon, acacia powder (if using), and cacao powder. Blend on high speed for 1 minute, until smooth.

Ingredient tip: You can order acacia powder online, but it may also be available in the grocery or health food store. Look for a good quality, organic variety and add 1 teaspoon to any smoothie recipe for a prebiotic boost.

Per Serving: Calories: 392; Total Fat: 18g; Saturated Fat: 2g; Cholesterol: 0mg; Carbohydrates: 50g; Fiber: 16g; Protein: 19g

Chocolate-Fig Smoothie

DAIRY-FREE, GLUTEN-FREE, NIGHTSHADE-FREE
SERVES 2 PREP TIME: 10 minutes

Not only does this smoothie taste like a chocolate milkshake, but it also contains cinnamon, which can help control blood sugar, and figs for better digestion. The kale adds important vitamins and minerals, such as magnesium, that many Americans lack in their diet. Magnesium is involved in more than 400 reactions in the body, so adequate intake is vital for your overall health.

2½ cups unsweetened nut or seed milk (almond, coconut, flax, or hemp seed)

2 cups chopped curly kale

1 cup frozen blueberries

½ frozen banana

1 fresh fig (see tip)

1 scoop vanilla collagen peptides (optional)

2 scoops vegan chocolate protein powder

2 tablespoons chia seeds

1 teaspoon ground cinnamon

2 teaspoons acacia powder (optional)

1½ teaspoons cacao powder

In a blender, combine the nut milk, kale, blueberries, banana, fig, collagen peptides (if using), protein powder, chia seeds, cinnamon, acacia powder (if using), and cacao powder. Blend on high speed for 1 minute, until smooth.

Ingredient tip: If you can't find fresh figs, use 1 or 2 dried figs, but know that the dried figs will increase the natural sugar content of the smoothie.

Per Serving: Calories: 372; Total Fat: 12g; Saturated Fat: 1g; Cholesterol: 0mg; Carbohydrates: 52g; Fiber: 19g; Protein: 26g

Berry-Peach Smoothie

DAIRY-FREE, GLUTEN-FREE, NIGHTSHADE-FREE
SERVES 2 **PREP TIME:** 10 minutes

Flaxseed is a great plant-based source of protein, and it contains powerful antioxidants such as lignans. In addition, flaxseed provides soluble and insoluble fiber to aid digestion and feed the gut microbiome. Dandelion greens are nutritious and mild in flavor, so they work well in smoothies.

2½ cups unsweetened nut or seed milk (almond, coconut, flax, or hemp seed)

2 tablespoons whole-milled flaxseed

2 cups dandelion greens, chopped

1 scoop vanilla collagen peptides (optional)

1 scoop vegan vanilla protein powder

½ teaspoon ground cinnamon

2 teaspoons acacia powder (optional)

½ cup frozen sliced peaches

1 cup frozen blueberries

In a blender, combine the nut milk, flaxseed, dandelion greens, collagen peptides (if using), protein powder, cinnamon, acacia powder (if using), peaches, and blueberries. Blend on high speed for 1 minute, until smooth.

> **Ingredient tip:** When buying flaxseed, choose ground or whole-milled varieties instead of whole flaxseed, which is difficult to digest. If you have difficulty finding fresh dandelion greens, substitute an equal amount of chopped kale or spinach.

Per Serving: Calories: 260; Total Fat: 8g; Saturated Fat: <1g; Cholesterol: 0mg; Carbohydrates: 37g; Fiber: 11g; Protein: 16g

Pineapple-Ginger Smoothie

DAIRY-FREE, GLUTEN-FREE, NIGHTSHADE-FREE

SERVES 2 PREP TIME: 10 minutes

This smoothie harnesses the anti-inflammatory power of fresh ginger with a refreshing tropical twist. The bioactive compound gingerol is responsible for ginger's anti-inflammatory and antioxidant effects, but the fresh root can also improve digestion. The chia seeds in this smoothie provide plenty of fiber and plant-based protein, as well as omega-3 fatty acids for even more anti-inflammatory benefits.

2½ cups unsweetened nut or seed milk (almond, coconut, flax, or hemp seed)

2 cups fresh spinach

1 celery stalk, coarsely chopped

2 tablespoons chia seeds

1 cup fresh pineapple chunks

1 tablespoon minced peeled fresh ginger

1 scoop vanilla collagen peptides (optional)

2 scoops vegan vanilla protein powder

½ frozen banana

In a blender, combine the nut milk, spinach, celery, chia seeds, pineapple, ginger, collagen peptides (if using), protein powder, and banana. Blend on high speed for 1 minute, until smooth.

> **Ingredient tip:** To prep fresh ginger, simply peel off the skin and mince the flesh, then add it to smoothies, marinades, and dressings. You can use ground ginger instead, although it may not provide the same benefits. For every 1 tablespoon of fresh ginger, substitute 1 teaspoon of ground ginger.

Per Serving: Calories: 334; Total Fat: 10g; Saturated Fat: <1g;

Cholesterol: 0mg; Carbohydrates: 43g; Fiber: 13g; Protein: 26g

Purple Cruciferous Berry Smoothie

DAIRY-FREE, GLUTEN-FREE, NIGHTSHADE-FREE, VEGAN

SERVES 2 **PREP TIME:** 10 minutes

Although red cabbage in a smoothie is a bit unusual, I promise you won't even know it's there. The tart berries and bananas make this smoothie a delicious way to reap the benefits of this powerful cruciferous vegetable. Loaded with vitamins C and K and fiber, this smoothie boosts healthy digestion and gut microbiome diversity—powerful drivers of health.

2½ cups unsweetened nut or seed milk (almond, coconut, flax, or hemp seed)

1 cup fresh spinach

1 small mini cucumber, sliced

1 cup shredded red cabbage

2 scoops vegan vanilla protein powder (optional)

1 teaspoon ground cinnamon

2 tablespoons whole-milled flaxseed

½ frozen banana

1 cup frozen blueberries

2 tablespoons almond butter or Pumpkin Seed Butter (page 127)

In a blender, combine the nut milk, spinach, cucumber, red cabbage, protein powder (if using), cinnamon, flaxseed, banana, blueberries, and almond butter. Blend on high speed for 1 minute until smooth.

Ingredient tip: To freeze fresh bananas, simply peel the bananas, break them into chunks, and place them in a freezer-safe container in the freezer for use in smoothie recipes or Creamy Cashew Milk Ice Cream (page 119).

Per Serving: Calories: 288; Total Fat: 16g; Saturated Fat: 1g; Cholesterol: 0mg; Carbohydrates: 35g; Fiber: 10g; Protein: 9g

Almond Butter and
Honey Overnight Oats

DAIRY-FREE, GLUTEN-FREE, NIGHTSHADE-FREE, VEGETARIAN
SERVES 5 PREP TIME: 15 minutes, plus 4 hours to chill

Uncooked oats are a great source of resistant starch to feed the gut microbiome. Although plain oats can leave you feeling hungry in the morning, this recipe includes plenty of healthy fat, fiber, and protein to keep you satisfied until lunch. It also calls for honey, a great source of antioxidant flavonoids and a prebiotic for gut bacteria.

1½ cups unsweetened nut or seed milk (almond, coconut, flax, or hemp seed)

1¼ cups certified gluten-free rolled oats

½ cup unsweetened coconut yogurt

¼ cup honey

¼ cup almond butter

¼ cup whole-milled flaxseed

1½ teaspoons vanilla extract

½ teaspoon sea salt

⅓ cup dried cranberries

¾ cup chopped walnuts

1. In a large bowl, stir together the nut milk, oats, yogurt, honey, almond butter, flax-seed, vanilla, and salt until well mixed. Divide the mixture among five half-pint jars and seal the lids. Refrigerate for at least 4 hours.

2. When ready to serve, open each jar and top with 1 tablespoon cranberries and about 2½ tablespoons walnuts.

Ingredient tip: Many commercially prepared nut but-ters contain inflammatory fats. Look for varieties with no added oils, or make your own Pumpkin Seed Butter (page 127) to use instead.

Per Serving: Calories: 406; Total Fat: 24g; Saturated Fat: 3g; Cholesterol: 0mg; Carbohydrates: 45g; Fiber: 7g; Protein: 10g

Blackberry-Walnut Breakfast Quinoa

DAIRY-FREE, GLUTEN-FREE, NIGHTSHADE-FREE, VEGETARIAN

SERVES 4 PREP TIME: 10 minutes **COOK TIME:** 20 minutes

You may not think of quinoa as a breakfast food, but this powerful seed is a complete source of protein in a plant-based form. It is also a good source of fiber and resistant starch to feed the gut microbiome, which can help lower inflammation in the body. Blackberries add color and a touch of sweetness to this dish, along with immune system–supporting vitamin C.

1 cup quinoa, rinsed well

1 cup water

1 cup unsweetened nut or seed milk (almond, coconut, flax, or hemp seed)

1 teaspoon ground cinnamon

1 teaspoon vanilla extract

½ cup dried cranberries

1 cup chopped walnuts

1 tablespoon honey

2 cups fresh blackberries

1. In a medium saucepan, stir together the quinoa, water, nut milk, cinnamon, and vanilla and bring to a boil. Reduce the heat to low, cover the pan, and simmer for about 15 minutes, or until the quinoa has absorbed the liquid. Remove the saucepan from the heat.

2. In a medium bowl, stir together the quinoa mixture, cranberries, walnuts, and honey until well combined.

3. Top each portion with ½ cup fresh blackberries and serve hot or cold.

Ingredient tip: Quinoa contains saponin, an outer coating with a bitter or soapy taste, so rinse quinoa before cooking it. Use a fine-mesh strainer and rinse the quinoa with cool water until the water runs clear, or buy prewashed quinoa.

Per Serving: Calories: 481; Total Fat: 23g; Saturated Fat: 2g; Cholesterol: 0mg; Carbohydrates: 63g; Fiber: 11g; Protein: 11g

Baked Cranberry-Pecan Oatmeal

DAIRY-FREE, GLUTEN-FREE, NIGHTSHADE-FREE, VEGAN
SERVES 6 PREP TIME: 10 minutes COOK TIME: 35 minutes

This hearty dish provides a healthy dose of resistant starch to keep your gut microbiome happy. Eating apples daily provides your gut microbiome with much needed prebiotic fiber. Apples also contain quercetin and vitamin C, which along with the fiber, are important for optimal immune system function.

3 cups unsweetened nut or seed milk (almond, coconut, flax, or hemp seed)

3 tablespoons coconut sugar

1½ tablespoons coconut oil

2 teaspoons ground cinnamon

1½ cups certified gluten-free rolled oats

1½ cups finely chopped apple (about 1 large)

¾ cup dried cranberries

¾ cup coarsely chopped pecans

1. Preheat the oven to 350°F. Line a 9-inch baking dish with parchment paper.

2. In a large saucepan, combine the nut milk, coconut sugar, coconut oil, and cinnamon and bring to a boil.

3. Meanwhile, in a large bowl, stir together the oats, apple, cranberries, and pecans. Spread the mixture evenly in the prepared baking dish.

4. When the milk mixture begins to boil, pour it over the oatmeal mixture.

5. Bake, uncovered, for 35 minutes, or until the liquid has been absorbed and the oatmeal is tender.

Variation tip: You can vary the flavor of this dish by changing the type of fruit you use. I like blueberries or blackberries in this dish, too.

Per Serving: Calories: 322; Total Fat: 16g; Saturated Fat: 4g; Cholesterol: 0mg; Carbohydrates: 45g; Fiber: 6g; Protein: 5g

Apple Breakfast Bowl

DAIRY-FREE, GLUTEN-FREE, NIGHTSHADE-FREE, VEGAN

SERVES 4 **PREP TIME:** 15 minutes

The apples and coconut yogurt in this breakfast bowl help boost normal immune system function. Coconut yogurt is a fermented food that can improve the balance in your gut microbiome. I like to use Gala apples for this recipe for their crisp flesh and mildly sweet flavor.

4 medium apples, diced

4 (6-ounce) containers unsweetened coconut yogurt

¼ cup whole-milled flaxseed

½ teaspoon ground cinnamon

In a medium bowl, stir together the apples, yogurt, flaxseed, and cinnamon.

Ingredient tip: Many coconut yogurts contain high amounts of sugar and additives, as well as inflammatory non nutritive sweeteners like sucralose and aspartame. Be sure to read the food labels and look for a fermented coconut yogurt with no added sugar.

Per Serving: Calories: 215; Total Fat: 8g; Saturated Fat: 5g; Cholesterol: 0mg; Carbohydrates: 36g; Fiber: 9g; Protein: 3g

Pumpkin-Flax Muffins

DAIRY-FREE, GLUTEN-FREE, NIGHTSHADE-FREE, VEGETARIAN
SERVES 6 PREP TIME: 10 minutes COOK TIME: 50 minutes

Pumpkin is a wonderful source of fiber, as well as vitamins A and C to strengthen the immune system. Take advantage of this powerhouse squash all year long by using canned pure pumpkin (not pumpkin pie filling). These muffins are savory; for a sweeter version, fold in ½ cup of dried cranberries.

6 tablespoons whole-milled flaxseed

1 (15-ounce) can pure pumpkin

½ cup coconut oil, melted

3 tablespoons honey

1 tablespoon pure maple syrup

½ teaspoon vanilla extract

1 teaspoon freshly squeezed lemon juice

½ cup coconut flour

½ teaspoon baking soda

½ teaspoon ground nutmeg

½ teaspoon ground cinnamon

½ cup chopped walnuts

1. Preheat the oven to 350°F. Line a 12-cup muffin tin with baking cups.

2. In a medium bowl, stir together the flaxseed and pumpkin until well combined.

3. Add the melted coconut oil, honey, maple syrup, vanilla, and lemon juice and mix well.

4. Add the coconut flour, baking soda, nutmeg, and cinnamon and mix to combine.

5. Fold in the chopped walnuts. Evenly divide the batter among the prepared muffin cups. Use the back of a spoon to gently press the batter evenly into the muffin cups.

6. Bake for 50 minutes, or until a toothpick inserted into the center of a muffin comes out clean. Let the muffins cool before serving.

7. Refrigerate leftovers in an airtight container for up to 5 days.

Batch cook tip: These muffins freeze well, so double the recipe and freeze them in individual servings for up to 3 months for a quick breakfast or snack.

Per Serving: Calories: 372; Total Fat: 28g; Saturated Fat: 17g;

Cholesterol: 0mg; Carbohydrates: 26g; Fiber: 8g; Protein: 5g

Root Vegetable Breakfast Skillet

DAIRY-FREE, GLUTEN-FREE, NIGHTSHADE-FREE, VEGAN
SERVES 4 PREP TIME: 10 minutes COOK TIME: 25 minutes

Root vegetables, such as purple-top turnips, are full of fiber to fuel the gut microbiome, and they also contain antioxidants, minerals, and vitamins to reduce inflammation in the fight against chronic inflammatory diseases such as psoriasis. This hearty breakfast is sure to keep your energy level steady and keep you full until lunch.

2 tablespoons avocado oil

1 cup diced yellow onion

4 garlic cloves, minced

⅔ cup chopped asparagus

⅔ cup diced carrot

2 cups cubed unpeeled sweet potato

2 cups cubed peeled purple-top turnip

¼ teaspoon sea salt

½ cup low-sodium vegetable broth

4 ounces fresh spinach (about 4 cups)

1. In a medium skillet over medium-high heat, combine the oil, onion, and garlic. Cook for 5 minutes, or until the onion is translucent and fragrant.

2. Add the asparagus and carrot and cook for about 8 minutes, or until tender.

3. Add the sweet potato, turnip, salt, and broth. Cover the skillet and cook over medium-high heat for about 10 minutes, or until the sweet potatoes and turnips are tender.

4. Add the spinach and cook for 2 minutes, or until wilted.

5. Divide the mixture evenly among four bowls and serve.

Substitution tip: If you tolerate nightshade vegetables, substitute red and yellow bell peppers in equal amounts for the asparagus and carrot for a change of pace.

Per Serving: Calories: 238; Total Fat: 7g; Saturated Fat: 1g; Cholesterol: 0mg; Carbohydrates: 41g; Fiber: 8g; Protein: 5g

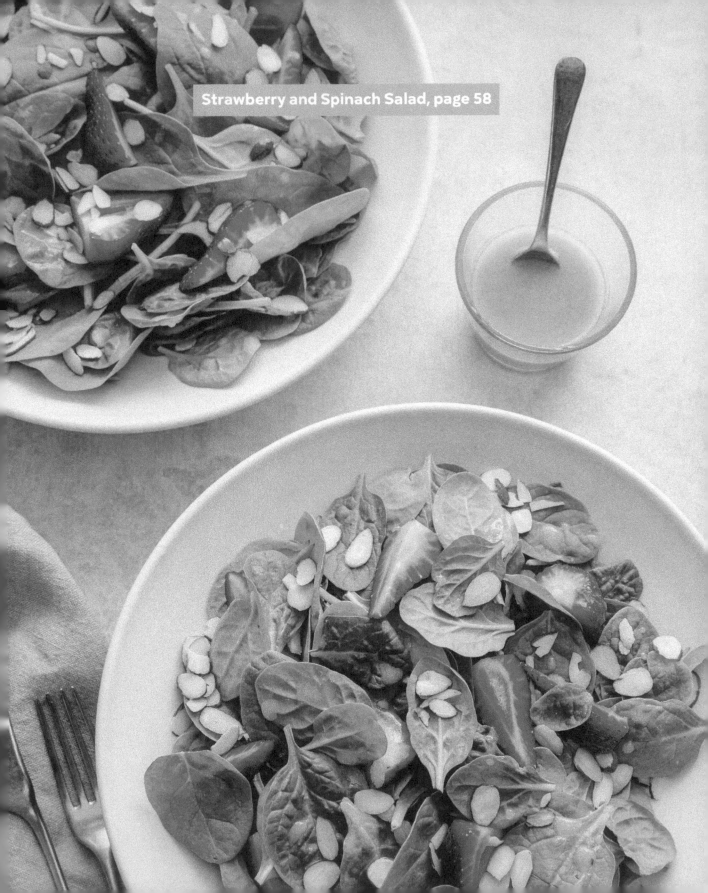

Strawberry and Spinach Salad, page 58

5
VEGETARIAN AND VEGAN

Colorful Bean and Nut Salad

DAIRY-FREE, GLUTEN-FREE, VEGETARIAN
SERVES 4 **PREP TIME:** 20 minutes

This festive salad makes a great entrée when served over a bed of fresh greens. The olive oil helps reduce inflammation in the body while enhancing immune function.

For the salad

1 (15-ounce) can pinto beans, drained and rinsed

1 (15-ounce) can cannellini beans, drained and rinsed

¼ cup extra-virgin olive oil

1 head broccoli, chopped

6 scallions, white and green parts, chopped

1 large red bell pepper, diced

2 medium carrots, grated

1 medium red onion, sliced

½ cup raw almonds, chopped

For the dressing

⅓ cup extra-virgin olive oil

¼ cup apple cider vinegar with the mother

2 tablespoons Dijon mustard

2 teaspoons honey

2 teaspoons dried basil

2 teaspoons dried oregano

½ teaspoon sea salt

¼ teaspoon freshly ground black pepper

1. **To make the salad:** In a large bowl, stir together the pinto beans, cannellini beans, and oil to coat.

2. Add the broccoli, scallions, bell pepper, carrots, and red onion to the beans and mix well.

3. **To make the dressing:** In a small, lidded mason jar or salad dressing shaker, combine the oil, vinegar, mustard, honey, basil, oregano, salt, and pepper. Seal the jar and shake well to combine. Pour the dressing over the salad and toss to coat well.

4. When ready to serve, sprinkle each serving with 2 tablespoons chopped almonds.

Substitution tip: If you don't tolerate nightshades, substitute ½ cup of chopped cauliflower for the red bell pepper.

Per Serving: Calories: 659; Total Fat: 42g; Saturated Fat: 5g; Cholesterol: 0mg; Carbohydrates: 57g; Fiber: 18g; Protein: 20g

Black Bean Salad with Creamy Avocado Dressing

GLUTEN-FREE, DAIRY-FREE, NIGHTSHADE-FREE, VEGETARIAN
SERVES 4 PREP TIME: 15 minutes

Avocados are very popular these days and for good reason. Not only are they high in anti-inflammatory monounsaturated fat, but they also contain an unbelievable amount of dietary fiber. Avocados are a great substitute for mayonnaise in dressings, but they brown quickly. To keep your dressing nice and green, store it with the removed avocado pit.

For the dressing

1½ avocados, peeled, halved, and pitted

½ small cucumber

1 scallion, white and green parts

1 tablespoon freshly squeezed lime juice

¼ cup extra-virgin olive oil

1 tablespoon apple cider vinegar with the mother

1 teaspoon honey

½ teaspoon dried dill weed

½ teaspoon dried basil

¼ teaspoon freshly ground black pepper

¼ teaspoon sea salt

For the salad

1 medium head green or red leaf lettuce, chopped

1 (15-ounce) can black beans, drained and rinsed

3 cups shredded red cabbage

2 cups chopped broccoli

1 medium cucumber, sliced with the skin on

½ medium red onion, thinly sliced

¼ cup whole shelled hemp seeds

1. **To make the dressing:** In a small food processor, combine the avocados, cucumber, scallion, lime juice, oil, vinegar, honey, dill, basil, pepper, and salt. Process until smooth.

2. **To make the salad:** In a large bowl, mix together the leaf lettuce, black beans, red cabbage, broccoli, cucumber, red onion, and hemp seeds.

3. Pour the dressing over the salad and toss well to coat and combine.

Ingredient tip: To store leftovers, keep the salad ingredients in separate containers and serve the dressing on the side to prevent the salad from getting soggy.

Per Serving: Calories: 433; Total Fat: 27g; Saturated Fat: 4g; Cholesterol: 0mg;

Carbohydrates: 40g; Fiber: 17g; Protein: 14g

Strawberry and Spinach Salad

GLUTEN-FREE, DAIRY-FREE, NIGHTSHADE-FREE, VEGETARIAN

SERVES 2 as an entrée, 4 as a side   **PREP TIME:** 10 minutes   **COOK TIME:** 20 minutes

Instead of croutons, which are high in inflammatory ingredients and gluten, this salad is topped with roasted almonds, pecans, and seeds. Nuts and seeds have a variety of anti-inflammatory polyunsaturated and monounsaturated fats as well as important minerals like magnesium and selenium. They can even act as a prebiotic for the gut and can help control blood sugar levels.

For the salad

1 cup certified gluten-free rolled oats

½ cup raw pecans

½ cup raw almonds

½ cup raw sunflower seeds

¼ cup raw pepitas (shelled pumpkin seeds)

¼ cup avocado oil

½ teaspoon sea salt

1 tablespoon pure maple syrup

6 cups fresh spinach, chopped

10 medium strawberries, hulled and sliced

1 large kohlrabi, peeled and diced

1 large avocado, peeled, halved, and pitted

For the dressing

3 tablespoons extra-virgin olive oil

2 tablespoons freshly squeezed lemon juice

1 tablespoon Dijon mustard

1 teaspoon honey

¼ teaspoon sea salt

⅛ teaspoon freshly ground black pepper

1. Preheat the oven to 350°F. Line a baking sheet with parchment paper.

2. **To make the salad:** In a medium bowl, stir together the oats, pecans, almonds, sunflower seeds, and pepitas.

3. Add the avocado oil, salt, and maple syrup to the oat mixture and stir to incorporate well. Spread the oat mixture on the prepared baking sheet in a single layer.

4. Bake for 10 minutes. Turn the baking sheet 180 degrees and bake for 7 minutes more, or until golden brown.

5. In a large bowl, combine the spinach, strawberries, and kohlrabi.

6. **To make the dressing:** In a small, lidded mason jar or salad shaker, combine the olive oil, lemon juice, mustard, honey, salt, and pepper. Seal the jar and shake well to combine.

7. **To finish the salad:** Top the spinach, strawberries, and kohlrabi with ½ cup of the oat and nut mixture and the dressing, and toss to coat well.

8. Top each entrée portion of salad with ½ avocado. If preparing as side salads, add ¼ avocado to each salad.

Make it easier: The nut mixture creates about 11 (¼-cup) servings, leaving you with 9 portions after making this recipe. The mixture will last for about 1 week in an airtight container and makes a great trail mix snack or a topping for other salads.

Per Serving: (entrée) Calories: 834; Total Fat: 68g; Saturated Fat: 9g; Cholesterol: 0mg; Carbohydrates: 50g; Fiber: 22g; Protein: 16g

Quinoa, Pomegranate, and Spinach Bowl

DAIRY-FREE, GLUTEN-FREE, NIGHTSHADE-FREE, VEGAN

SERVES 4 PREP TIME: 20 minutes

This all-in-one bowl combines greens and fermented foods to fuel the gut microbiome and walnuts as a source of healthy fat. But the real star of this recipe is the pomegranate. The fruit contains powerful polyphenols called ellagitannins, which have strong anticancer, anti-inflammatory, and antioxidant effects. It can also decrease inflammation in the digestive tract and throughout the body.

For the salad

2 cups cooked quinoa

6 cups fresh spinach

½ cup fresh pomegranate arils

1 avocado, peeled, halved, pitted, and diced

½ cup chopped walnuts

For the dressing

2 tablespoons apple cider vinegar with the mother

1½ tablespoons extra-virgin olive oil

1 tablespoon freshly squeezed lemon juice

1 garlic clove, minced

¼ teaspoon dried basil

⅛ teaspoon sea salt

⅛ teaspoon freshly ground black pepper

1. **To make the salad:** In a large bowl, toss together the cooked quinoa, spinach, pomegranate arils, avocado, and walnuts.

2. **To make the dressing:** In a small, lidded mason jar or salad dressing shaker, combine the vinegar, oil, lemon juice, garlic, basil, salt, and pepper. Seal the jar and shake well to combine. Pour the dressing over the salad and toss to coat and combine.

Make it easier: This recipe comes together quickly, but to make it even more of a breeze, prepare the dressing up to 3 days ahead and refrigerate in an airtight container for up to 5 days.

Per Serving: Calories: 340; Total Fat: 22g; Saturated Fat: 3g; Cholesterol: 0mg; Carbohydrates: 31g; Fiber: 8g; Protein: 9g

Easy Vegan Hummus Bowl

DAIRY-FREE, GLUTEN-FREE, NIGHTSHADE-FREE, VEGAN

SERVES 4 **PREP TIME:** 15 minutes

Hummus makes a versatile snack, but it can also make a great vegan or vegetarian plant-based entrée for lunch or dinner. This simple bowl is loaded with protein and anti-inflammatory nutrients. It also has an incredible amount of fiber from the avocado, beans, and spinach to fuel your gut microbiome.

8 cups fresh baby spinach

1 cup Savory Sweet Potato Hummus (page 125)

1 medium carrot, grated

1 cup canned cannellini beans, drained and rinsed

½ cup Simple Italian Salad Dressing (page 132)

1 cup dry-roasted cashews, chopped

2 medium avocados, peeled, halved, pitted, and sliced

1. To assemble each bowl, combine 2 cups spinach, ¼ cup sweet potato hummus, one-fourth of the grated carrot, and ¼ cup cannellini beans in each bowl.

2. Drizzle each portion with 2 tablespoons dressing.

3. Top each bowl with ¼ cup cashews and slices from ½ avocado.

Make-ahead tip: This is the perfect lunch bowl for busy work days. Simply prep your hummus bowls ahead of time and leave the dressing and avocado on the side. You can refrigerate it, covered, for up to 3 days.

Per Serving: Calories: 686; Total Fat: 57g; Saturated Fat: 9g; Cholesterol: 0mg; Carbohydrates: 38g; Fiber: 12g; Protein: 14g

Mushroom-Zucchini Sauté

GLUTEN-FREE, DAIRY-FREE, NIGHTSHADE-FREE, VEGAN

SERVES 4 PREP TIME: 10 minutes COOK TIME: 15 minutes

An anti-inflammatory powerhouse, mushrooms add a meaty texture to this satisfying sauté. Mushrooms contain beta-glucans, a type of soluble fiber that can be helpful for maintaining a healthy gut microbiome. They also happen to be one of only a few good food sources of vitamin D. Inadequate vitamin D levels are common in those with autoimmune diseases such as psoriasis, so it's wise to seek out foods high in this vitamin.

¼ cup avocado oil

4 garlic cloves, minced

1 pound baby bella mushrooms, thinly sliced

2 medium zucchini, sliced

½ cup chopped fresh basil

2 tablespoons balsamic vinegar

2 tablespoons freshly squeezed lemon juice

8 cups arugula

4 tablespoons extra-virgin olive oil

6 tablespoons whole shelled hemp seeds

1. In a large skillet over medium heat, heat the avocado oil. Add the garlic and sauté for 2 minutes. Add the mushrooms and zucchini and sauté for 10 minutes, or until the vegetables are softened.

2. Stir in the basil, vinegar, and lemon juice. Sauté for 2 minutes.

3. Divide the arugula among four bowls and drizzle each serving with 1 tablespoon olive oil.

4. Add equal portions of the mushroom and zucchini mixture to each bowl and top each with 1½ tablespoons hemp seeds.

Substitution tip: To boost the probiotic effect of this dish, use apple cider vinegar with the mother instead of balsamic vinegar.

Per Serving: Calories: 389; Total Fat: 35g; Saturated Fat: 4g; Cholesterol: 0mg; Carbohydrates: 14g; Fiber: 3g; Protein: 10g

Leek and Kohlrabi Stir-Fry

DAIRY-FREE, GLUTEN-FREE, NIGHTSHADE-FREE, VEGAN
SERVES 6 **PREP TIME:** 20 minutes **COOK TIME:** 15 minutes

This recipe highlights two powerful vegetables to include every week in your meal plan. Leeks—in the garlic and onion family—act as a prebiotic to maintain gut microbiome health. Kohlrabi, a member of the cabbage family, is high in fiber, and it also boasts a variety of antioxidants including anthocyanins, glucosinolates, and vitamin C to support immune function and prevent chronic disease.

2 tablespoons avocado oil

2 garlic cloves, minced

4 cups chopped well-cleaned leeks (about 4 medium leeks; see tip)

2 medium kohlrabi, peeled and chopped

2 (15-ounce) cans chickpeas, drained and rinsed

½ teaspoon sea salt

¼ teaspoon freshly ground black pepper

½ teaspoon ground coriander

6 cups Swiss chard, chopped

6 tablespoons extra-virgin olive oil

2 tablespoons balsamic vinegar

2 cups cooked quinoa

1. In a large wok or skillet over medium heat, combine the avocado oil, garlic, leeks, and kohlrabi. Sauté for about 8 minutes, or until browned.

2. Stir in the chickpeas, salt, pepper, and coriander and cook for 5 minutes, or until fragrant and the chickpeas are softened.

3. Meanwhile, in a large salad bowl, toss together the Swiss chard, olive oil, and vinegar.

4. Add the cooked quinoa and leeks and kohlrabi to the salad and mix well.

Ingredient tip: To prepare leeks, trim off the root end and cut the white and light green parts into rings. Soak the rings in cold water and let the dirt between the layers sink to the bottom. Lift the rings from the water using your hands (to leave the sediment on the bottom) and transfer to a fine-mesh strainer to drain.

Per Serving: Calories: 418; Total Fat: 22g; Saturated Fat: 3g; Cholesterol: 0mg; Carbohydrates: 47g; Fiber: 11g; Protein: 11g

White Bean and Cauliflower Skillet

GLUTEN-FREE, DAIRY-FREE, NIGHTSHADE-FREE, VEGAN

SERVES 6 PREP TIME: 15 minutes COOK TIME: 20 minutes

Leafy greens are foundational for building a healthy gut microbiome. The arugula in this recipe is a cruciferous vegetable and it offers a slightly spicy bite. Like other greens, arugula is high in fiber; vitamins A, C, and K; folate; and potassium. Try to eat at least three servings of greens (1 cup cooked or ½ cup raw) every day to promote gut microbiome diversity.

2 tablespoons coconut oil

2 garlic cloves, chopped

1 medium yellow onion, diced

1 large head cauliflower, coarsely chopped

2 (15-ounce) cans great northern beans, drained and rinsed

1½ teaspoons dried thyme

1½ teaspoons dried oregano

3 tablespoons water

1 teaspoon sea salt

½ teaspoon freshly ground black pepper

9 cups arugula

3 tablespoons extra-virgin olive oil

6 tablespoons whole shelled hemp seeds

1. In a large cast-iron skillet or wok over medium-high heat, heat the coconut oil. Add the garlic and cook for 1 to 2 minutes, stirring.

2. Add the onion and cauliflower and cook for about 10 minutes, until softened and browned.

3. Stir in the beans, thyme, oregano, water, salt, and pepper. Cover the skillet and cook for 5 minutes.

4. Stir in the arugula and cook for 3 minutes, or until wilted.

5. Drizzle each serving with 1½ teaspoons olive oil and sprinkle with 1 tablespoon hemp seeds.

Variation tip: For a heartier meal, serve over ½ cup of cooked quinoa.

Per Serving: Calories: 352; Total Fat: 17g; Saturated Fat: 6g; Cholesterol: 0mg; Carbohydrates: 37g; Fiber: 11g; Protein: 17g

Savory Seasoned Beans

DAIRY-FREE, GLUTEN-FREE, NIGHTSHADE-FREE, VEGAN

SERVES 4 **PREP TIME:** 10 minutes **COOK TIME:** 20 minutes

These seasoned beans are a staple at our house because they are full of flavor and simple to make. Beans provide valuable fiber and resistant starch for maintaining a healthy gut. They also provide protein and minerals, plus they offer antioxidant benefits. This tasty, versatile bean dish works great as a side dish, salad topper, or entrée.

3 tablespoons avocado oil

2 garlic cloves, chopped

1 medium yellow onion, chopped

1 (15-ounce) can black beans, drained and rinsed

1 (15-ounce) can great northern beans, drained and rinsed

2 tablespoons water

1 tablespoon ground cumin

1½ teaspoons ground coriander

1 teaspoon dried basil

½ teaspoon sea salt

¼ teaspoon freshly ground black pepper

1. In a large skillet over medium heat, combine the oil and garlic and sauté for 2 minutes.

2. Add the onion and sauté for 5 minutes.

3. Stir in the black beans and great northern beans and cook for 5 minutes.

4. Stir in the water, cumin, coriander, basil, salt, and pepper. Cover the skillet and cook for 5 minutes, or until the flavors are incorporated and the beans are soft.

Ingredient tip: When buying canned beans, look for nongenetically modified options that are packed in cans with BPA-free liners. BPA, or bisphenol A, is a hormone disrupter that's been linked to metabolic diseases such as obesity and type 2 diabetes.

Per Serving: Calories: 323; Total Fat: 11g; Saturated Fat: 1g; Cholesterol: 0mg; Carbohydrates: 43g; Fiber: 14g; Protein: 15g

Turnip and Greens Soup

DAIRY-FREE, GLUTEN-FREE, NIGHTSHADE-FREE, VEGAN

SERVES 6 **PREP TIME:** 15 minutes **COOK TIME:** 40 minutes

This one-pot recipe features two powerful anti-inflammatory vegetables: purple-top turnips and Swiss chard. Turnips are high in vitamin C, which supports a healthy immune system, and they also contain flavonoids and glucosinolates, powerful antioxidants for disease prevention. Swiss chard is full of flavonoids; vitamins A, C, and K; and the mineral magnesium.

¼ cup avocado oil

2 garlic cloves, minced

2 medium carrots, chopped

2 celery stalks, chopped

1 medium yellow onion, diced

4 medium purple-top turnips, peeled and cubed

1 yellow squash, cubed

6 cups low-sodium vegetable broth

2 dried bay leaves

1 teaspoon dried oregano

½ teaspoon dried thyme

½ teaspoon ground coriander

½ teaspoon celery salt

½ teaspoon sea salt

¼ teaspoon freshly ground black pepper

½ cup dried green lentils

2 cups chopped Swiss chard

1. In a large stockpot over medium heat, combine the oil, garlic, carrots, celery, and onion. Cook for about 5 minutes, or until softened.

2. Add the turnips and yellow squash and sauté for about 8 minutes, until softened.

3. Add the broth, bay leaves, oregano, thyme, coriander, celery salt, sea salt, and pepper. Increase the heat to high and bring the soup to a boil.

4. Add the lentils. Reduce the heat to medium, cover the pot, and cook for 20 minutes, or until the lentils are soft.

5. Stir in the Swiss chard and let wilt for about 5 minutes before serving.

Batch cook tip: Double this recipe and freeze the leftovers in freezer-safe containers for up to 3 months. To reheat, heat in a small saucepan over medium heat for 10 minutes.

Per Serving: Calories: 195; Total Fat: 10g; Saturated Fat: 1g; Cholesterol: 0mg; Carbohydrates: 23g; Fiber: 5g; Protein: 6g

Black Bean Soup

DAIRY-FREE, GLUTEN-FREE, NIGHTSHADE-FREE, VEGAN

SERVES 4 **PREP TIME:** 10 minutes **COOK TIME:** 25 minutes

When it comes to fueling good gut bacteria, there's no better option than beans. They're a great source of fiber and resistant starch, as well as an inexpensive source of protein for vegans and vegetarians. This simple Black Bean Soup is the perfect dinner side, but it is also a filling lunch option. If you're not accustomed to eating beans, there may be an increase in gas with this dish until your gut microbiome has time to adjust.

1 tablespoon coconut oil

1 medium red onion, chopped

4 garlic cloves, minced

2 (15-ounce) cans black beans, drained and rinsed

4 cups low-sodium vegetable broth

1 tablespoon ground cumin

½ teaspoon ground coriander

½ teaspoon sea salt

¼ teaspoon freshly ground black pepper

½ cup chopped scallions, white and green parts

1. In a large Dutch oven or stockpot over medium-high heat, combine the coconut oil and red onion and sauté for 3 minutes.

2. Add the garlic and sauté for another minute.

3. Stir in the black beans, broth, cumin, coriander, salt, and pepper. Increase the heat to high and bring the soup to a boil. Reduce the heat to medium-low and simmer the soup for 15 minutes.

4. To serve, add a sprinkle of scallions to each bowl.

Batch cook tip: This soup freezes well, so double the recipe and freeze in individual airtight containers for up to 3 months for a quick, healthy meal option.

Per Serving: Calories: 277; Total Fat: 5g; Saturated Fat: 3g; Cholesterol: 0mg; Carbohydrates: 46g; Fiber: 17g; Protein: 14g

Anti-Inflammatory Curry Stew

DAIRY-FREE, GLUTEN-FREE, NIGHTSHADE-FREE, VEGAN
SERVES 4 PREP TIME: 15 minutes COOK TIME: 45 minutes

Turmeric has traditionally been used for its unique flavor and medicinal benefits. The active compound in turmeric is curcumin, which is responsible for its anti-inflammatory and antioxidant capacity. Many store-bought curry powders contain nightshade spices. To make your own nightshade-free curry powder, combine 1 teaspoon each of ground turmeric, ground cumin, ground coriander, ground ginger, and dry mustard and ¼ teaspoon each of ground cinnamon and black pepper. This makes about 2 tablespoons. Save the leftovers in an airtight container for Spice-Rubbed Chicken Breast (page 102) or Curried Spaghetti Squash Shrimp (page 77).

2 tablespoons coconut oil

2 large yellow onions, diced

3 garlic cloves, minced

4 medium carrots, sliced

2 medium parsnips, unpeeled and diced

2 cups water

1 small head cauliflower, cut into small pieces

1 bunch baby bok choy, chopped

1 (14.5-ounce) can low-sodium green beans, drained and rinsed

3 teaspoons minced peeled fresh ginger

2 teaspoons nightshade-free curry powder (see headnote)

3 teaspoons ground turmeric

1 (15-ounce) can "lite" coconut milk

½ teaspoon sea salt

¼ teaspoon freshly ground black pepper

1. In a large stockpot over medium heat, combine the coconut oil and onions and sauté for 4 minutes.

2. Add the garlic and sauté for another minute.

3. Add the carrots, parsnips, and water. Simmer for about 10 minutes.

4. Stir in the cauliflower, bok choy, green beans, ginger, curry powder, and turmeric. Cover the pot and simmer the soup for 15 minutes.

5. Add the coconut milk, salt, and pepper and mix well. Reduce the heat to low and simmer for 10 minutes more, until the vegetables are soft.

Per Serving: Calories: 283; Total Fat: 14g; Saturated Fat: 11g;

Cholesterol: 9mg; Carbohydrates: 37g; Fiber: 10g; Protein: 7g

Spiced Falafel Balls

DAIRY-FREE, GLUTEN-FREE, NIGHTSHADE-FREE, VEGAN
SERVES 4 PREP TIME: 10 minutes, plus 30 minutes to chill COOK TIME: 10 minutes

Traditional falafel is deep-fried in unhealthy oils, which can promote inflammation in the body. This panfried version is just as delicious and offers the nutritional benefits of chickpeas, including fiber to fuel the gut microbiome and plant-based protein. The fresh mint enhances the flavor of this dish while stimulating digestion. When preparing these falafel balls, keep your hands wet, as there is no binder and the mixture can become crumbly, making panfrying difficult. Do not skip the chill time, as the mixture will be too crumbly to work with otherwise.

2 (15-ounce) cans chickpeas, drained and rinsed

2 garlic cloves, minced

2 tablespoons dried parsley

2 tablespoons ground coriander

2 tablespoons chopped fresh mint

2 teaspoons ground cumin

¼ cup gluten-free oat flour

2 teaspoons sea salt

½ teaspoon freshly ground black pepper

½ cup avocado oil

1. Line a small baking sheet with parchment paper.

2. Put the chickpeas in a food processor and process for about 30 seconds, until smooth.

3. Add the garlic, parsley, coriander, mint, cumin, oat flour, salt, and pepper and pulse until the ingredients are incorporated.

4. Using wet hands, shape the chickpea mixture into 16 equal-size balls and place on the prepared baking sheet in a single layer. Chill in the refrigerator for 30 minutes.

5. In a medium skillet over medium-high heat, heat the oil. Add the falafel balls and panfry for a total of 8 minutes, turning frequently.

Make it easier: This recipe makes plenty of falafel, so plan to have some for lunch or dinner the next day. I love serving these as a topper to the Carrot Salad with Spicy Greens (page 124).

Per Serving: Calories: 466; Total Fat: 32g; Saturated Fat: 4g; Cholesterol: 0mg; Carbohydrates: 37g; Fiber: 10g; Protein: 11g

Crispy Lentil Burgers

DAIRY-FREE, GLUTEN-FREE, NIGHTSHADE-FREE, VEGAN

SERVES 4 **PREP TIME:** 15 minutes **COOK TIME:** 40 minutes

Prepackaged plant-based "burgers" are often loaded with inflammatory fats and additives. These lentil burgers are a wholesome option and loaded with important nutrients found in mushrooms and, of course, the powerful lentil! Lentils are a great plant-based source of protein and are also high in fiber and provide B vitamins, iron, and magnesium.

1 tablespoon whole-milled flaxseed

3 tablespoons water

1 cup cooked brown or green lentils

¼ cup sunflower seeds

1 cup chopped baby bella mushrooms

¼ cup gluten-free oat flour

2 garlic cloves, minced

½ small red onion, chopped

1 tablespoon extra-virgin olive oil

1 teaspoon ground cumin

½ teaspoon sea salt

¼ teaspoon freshly ground black pepper

1. Preheat the oven to 350°F. Line a baking sheet with parchment paper.

2. In a small bowl, make a flax "egg" by stirring together the flaxseed and water. Let sit for 10 minutes to thicken.

3. In the meantime, in a food processor, combine the cooked lentils, sunflower seeds, mushrooms, oat flour, garlic, red onion, oil, cumin, salt, and pepper.

4. Once the flax "egg" mixture is thickened, add it to the food processor. Process on high speed for about 30 seconds, stopping to scrape down the sides of the food processer bowl several times. Transfer the mixture to a large bowl. Using your hands, form the mixture into 4 patties and place them on the prepared baking sheet.

5. Bake for 40 minutes, flipping halfway through the baking time, until golden brown.

Ingredient tip: The flax "egg" is a great substitute for a regular egg. To use as a substitute for 1 whole egg, simply mix 1 tablespoon of whole-milled flaxseed with 3 tablespoons of warm water and let sit for 10 minutes.

Per Serving: Calories: 188; Total Fat: 9g; Saturated Fat: 1g; Cholesterol: 0mg; Carbohydrates: 20g; Fiber: 5g; Protein: 8g

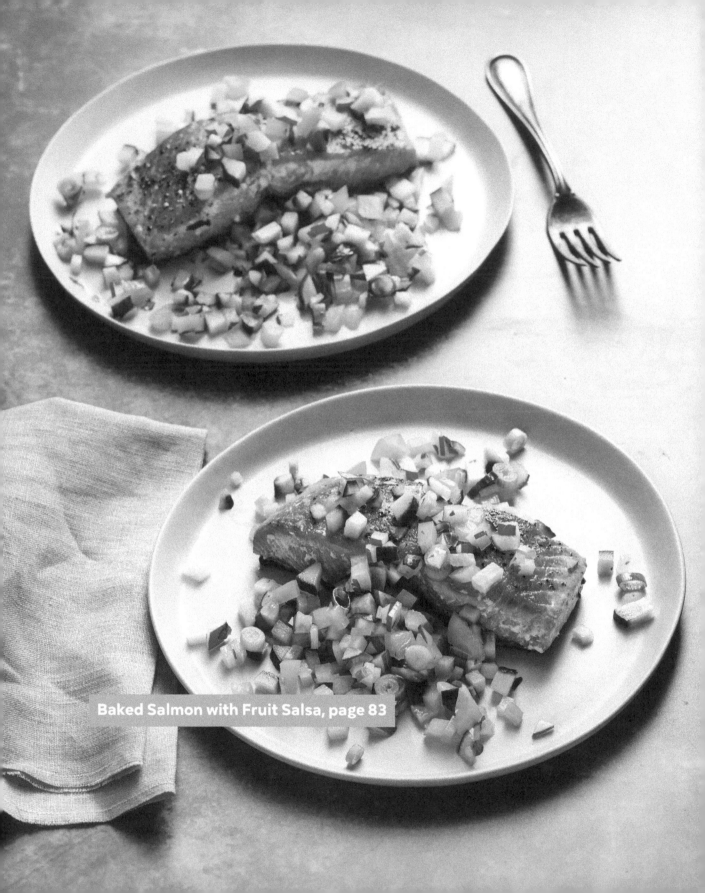

Baked Salmon with Fruit Salsa, page 83

6
FISH AND SEAFOOD

Mediterranean Tuna Salad

DAIRY-FREE, GLUTEN-FREE, NIGHTSHADE-FREE
SERVES 4 PREP TIME: 15 minutes

This simple but refreshing tuna salad is packed with lean protein and leafy greens to fuel your gut microbiome. The olives add monounsaturated fats and vitamin E to protect the body from oxidative damage. If you tolerate nightshades, try adding some cherry tomatoes to brighten up this dish.

8 cups mixed greens (arugula, baby spinach, and kale)

1 (15-ounce) can chickpeas, drained and rinsed

½ medium red onion, sliced

1 medium cucumber, diced with skin on

⅔ cup Simple Italian Salad Dressing (page 132)

2 (5-ounce) cans water-packed tuna, drained

1 ripe avocado, peeled, halved, pitted, and quartered

20 green olives, pitted

4 tablespoons whole shelled hemp seeds

1. In a large bowl, combine the greens, chickpeas, red onion, cucumber, salad dressing, and tuna. Mix until well combined and coated with the dressing.

2. Evenly divide the salad among four bowls, about 3 cups in each, and top each serving with 1 piece avocado, 5 olives, and 1 tablespoon hemp seeds.

Ingredient tip: Although tuna is high in omega-3 fats, it can also be high in mercury. Look for high quality, sustainable varieties such as albacore from the Pacific Northwest or northeast Pacific Ocean and skipjack from the Pacific Northwest or the eastern central Pacific Ocean.

Per Serving: Calories: 626; Total Fat: 49g; Saturated Fat: 7g; Cholesterol: 23mg; Carbohydrates: 28g; Fiber: 11g; Protein: 24g

Tuna Lettuce Wraps

GLUTEN-FREE, DAIRY-FREE, NIGHTSHADE-FREE
SERVES 4 PREP TIME: 15 minutes

A great lunch or light dinner option, these wraps contain two inflammation-fighting super-stars: omega-3-rich tuna and extra-virgin olive oil, which is full of monounsaturated fats and antioxidants. People who consume olive oil regularly tend to have lower rates of chronic inflammatory diseases. Serve with a side of Anti-Inflammatory Cauliflower Soup (page 122).

2 (5-ounce) cans water-packed tuna, drained

½ cup diced celery

½ cup chopped scallions, white and green parts

½ cup shredded carrots (about 1 medium)

¼ cup extra-virgin olive oil

1 tablespoon freshly squeezed lime juice

1 tablespoon Dijon mustard

1 teaspoon dill weed

½ teaspoon sea salt

¼ teaspoon freshly ground black pepper

8 butter lettuce leaves

1. In a large bowl, stir together the tuna, celery, scallions, and carrots.

2. In a small, lidded mason jar or salad dressing shaker, combine the oil, lime juice, mustard, dill, salt, and pepper. Seal the jar and shake well to combine. Pour the dressing over the tuna salad and mix until combined and coated.

3. Add ¼ cup tuna salad to each butter lettuce leaf and roll into a wrap.

Substitution tip: To add even more fiber to benefit your gut microbiome, substitute 8 collard or Swiss chard leaves for the butter lettuce leaves.

Per Serving: Calories: 194; Total Fat: 15g; Saturated Fat: 2g; Cholesterol: 23mg; Carbohydrates: 4g; Fiber: 1g; Protein: 13g

Baked Shrimp Veggie Packets

GLUTEN-FREE, DAIRY-FREE, NIGHTSHADE-FREE
SERVES 4 PREP TIME: 15 minutes COOK TIME: 15 minutes

Shrimp contains omega-3 fats, the mineral selenium, and the antioxidant carotenoid astaxanthin, which are important for fighting inflammation. The black pepper boosts the anti-inflammatory benefits of turmeric by making it more easily absorbed by the body.

¼ cup avocado oil

2 teaspoons Dijon mustard

1 teaspoon honey

1 teaspoon dried parsley

½ teaspoon ground turmeric

20 medium shrimp, peeled, deveined, and tails removed

1 large yellow onion, cut into thin rounds

½ teaspoon sea salt

¼ teaspoon freshly ground black pepper

8 cups chopped Swiss chard

1. Preheat the oven to 450°F.

2. Cut four large (about 11-by-16-inch) sheets of parchment paper.

3. In a medium bowl, whisk the oil, mustard, honey, parsley, and turmeric to blend. Add the shrimp to the bowl and toss well to coat.

4. To make the packets, fold each piece of parchment paper in half and then open back up. In the middle of each parchment square, place one-fourth of the onion slices as the bottom layer. Sprinkle with salt and pepper.

5. Add 2 cups Swiss chard on top of the onion layer in each packet.

6. Place 5 shrimp on top of the Swiss chard in each packet. Close the parchment packets by creating tight folds to seal. Place the packets on a baking sheet.

7. Bake for 15 minutes, or until the shrimp are opaque and reach an internal temperature of 145°F.

8. Open each packet slowly to allow steam to escape, then transfer the onion, greens, and shrimp to plates to serve.

Per Serving: Calories: 199; Total Fat: 15g; Saturated Fat: 2g;
Cholesterol: 77mg; Carbohydrates: 8g; Fiber: 2g; Protein: 10g

Curried Spaghetti Squash Shrimp

GLUTEN-FREE, DAIRY-FREE, NIGHTSHADE-FREE
SERVES 4 PREP TIME: 1 hour COOK TIME: 50 minutes

Avoiding refined grains can help lower inflammation in the body. Spaghetti squash is a wonderful gluten-free pasta alternative to refined grains, and it contains fiber, vitamins A, C, and K. The nightshade-free curry in this recipe helps target inflammation.

3 tablespoons avocado oil, divided

1 large spaghetti squash, halved and seeded

3 garlic cloves, minced

1 medium yellow onion, chopped

½ cup "lite" coconut milk

3 teaspoons nightshade-free curry powder (see Anti-Inflammatory Curry Stew page 68).

½ teaspoon sea salt

16 large shrimp, peeled and deveined

4 cups fresh baby spinach

1. Preheat the oven to 400°F. Line a baking sheet with parchment paper.

2. Drizzle 2 tablespoons oil over the flesh of both spaghetti squash halves and place the halves on the prepared baking sheet, flesh-side down.

3. Bake for 45 minutes, or until tender.

4. Meanwhile, in a large skillet or wok over medium heat, heat the remaining 1 tablespoon oil. Add the garlic and onion and sauté for 3 minutes.

5. Add the coconut milk, curry powder, salt, and shrimp to the skillet. Cook for 5 minutes, or until the shrimp are opaque and reach an internal temperature of 145°F.

6. When the spaghetti squash is done, remove it from the oven and, using a fork, scrape the flesh into strands.

7. Add the baby spinach and spaghetti squash to the skillet and mix well. Cook for about 5 minutes, until the spinach is wilted.

Make it easier: Bake the spaghetti squash and scrape the flesh the day before serving and refrigerate overnight.

Per Serving: Calories: 218; Total Fat: 13g; Saturated Fat: 3g;

Cholesterol: 61mg; Carbohydrates: 19g; Fiber: 5g; Protein: 10g

Baked Tilapia with Turmeric Sauce

GLUTEN-FREE, DAIRY-FREE, NIGHTSHADE-FREE
SERVES 4 **PREP TIME:** 5 minutes **COOK TIME:** 15 minutes

Although it contains less omega-3 fatty acids than other types of fish, tilapia is a great source of protein. It also contains niacin, selenium, and vitamin B_{12}. The turmeric and ginger in this recipe add an earthy, spicy flavor, in addition to their powerful anti-inflammatory and antioxidant benefits.

½ cup "lite" coconut milk

1 teaspoon ground turmeric

1 teaspoon ground cumin

1 teaspoon garlic powder

½ teaspoon sea salt

¼ teaspoon freshly ground black pepper

1 teaspoon minced peeled fresh ginger

2 garlic cloves, minced

4 (6-ounce) tilapia fillets

1. Preheat the oven to 425°F. Line a 9-by-13-inch baking dish with parchment paper.

2. In a small bowl, whisk the coconut milk, turmeric, cumin, garlic powder, salt, pepper, ginger, and garlic to combine.

3. Place the tilapia fillets in the prepared baking dish and pour the coconut milk mixture over the fish.

4. Bake for 15 minutes, or until the tilapia reaches an internal temperature of 145°F and flakes easily with a fork.

Ingredient tip: It is best to avoid tilapia sourced from China, due to concerns about farming practices, and to avoid farm-raised tilapia in general. If you have trouble finding sustainably sourced tilapia, substitute an equal amount of salmon or tuna in this recipe.

Per Serving: Calories: 225; Total Fat: 8g; Saturated Fat: 6g; Cholesterol: 85mg; Carbohydrates: 4g; Fiber: 1g; Protein: 35g

Nut and Oat–Crusted Cod

DAIRY-FREE, GLUTEN-FREE, NIGHTSHADE-FREE

SERVES 4 PREP TIME: 10 minutes **COOK TIME:** 15 minutes

Cod is a mild-tasting fish that's high in protein, selenium, and vitamin B_{12}. Cod is also lower in mercury compared to other varieties of fish. Walnuts contain omega-3 fats in the form of alpha-linolenic acid (ALA). Walnuts also have polyphenols and antioxidants to control blood sugar levels, increase beneficial bacteria in the gut, and decrease chronic disease risk. For a complete meal, pair this delicious cod with Simple Roasted Vegetables (page 126).

4 (6-ounce) cod fillets

½ teaspoon sea salt

½ teaspoon freshly ground black pepper

¼ cup gluten-free oat flour

½ cup walnuts, chopped

¼ cup extra-virgin olive oil

1. Preheat the oven to 400°F. Line a baking sheet with parchment paper.

2. Place the cod fillets on the prepared baking sheet and sprinkle each with salt and pepper.

3. In a small bowl, stir together the oat flour, walnuts, and oil until well combined. Spoon equal amounts of the nut mixture onto each cod fillet.

4. Bake for 15 minutes, or until the cod reaches an internal temperature of 145°F and flakes easily with a fork.

Ingredient tip: Cod is a versatile fish and can be baked, steamed, broiled, or used in stews or soups. However, Atlantic cod has been overfished, so it's important to look for a quality cod from sustainable sources.

Per Serving: Calories: 373; Total Fat: 25g; Saturated Fat: 3g;

Cholesterol: 88mg; Carbohydrates: 7g; Fiber: 2g; Protein: 33g

Tangy Cod with Brussels Sprouts and Rutabaga

GLUTEN-FREE, DAIRY-FREE, NIGHTSHADE-FREE

SERVES 4 PREP TIME: 15 minutes COOK TIME: 35 minutes

This sheet-pan dinner combines the delicate flavors of cod with two cruciferous vegetables: rutabaga and Brussels sprouts. Both contain glucosinolates, which are helpful for lowering inflammation in the body. They also contain vitamin C to support a healthy immune system.

3 large rutabagas, peeled and cut into chunks

1 medium red onion, quartered

1 pound Brussels sprouts, trimmed and halved

3 tablespoons plus 1 teaspoon avocado oil, divided

1 teaspoon sea salt, divided

½ teaspoon freshly ground black pepper, divided

4 teaspoons Dijon mustard

4 (6-ounce) cod fillets

1. Preheat the oven to 450°F. Line a sheet pan with parchment paper.

2. In a large bowl, toss together the rutabagas, red onion, Brussels sprouts, 2 tablespoons oil, ½ teaspoon salt, and ¼ teaspoon pepper until well mixed. Spread the vegetable mixture on the prepared sheet pan in a single layer.

3. Bake for 20 minutes.

4. Meanwhile, in a small bowl, whisk the mustard, remaining 1 tablespoon plus 1 teaspoon oil, remaining ½ teaspoon salt, and remaining ¼ teaspoon pepper until well mixed. Spoon an equal amount of the mustard mixture to the top of each piece of cod and brush to coat evenly.

5. When the rutabaga mixture has baked for 20 minutes, make room on the baking sheet and arrange the cod fillets among the vegetables.

6. Return the baking sheet to the oven and bake for 15 minutes more, or until the cod reaches an internal temperature of 145°F and flakes easily with a fork.

Per Serving: Calories: 509; Total Fat: 14g; Saturated Fat: 2g;

Cholesterol: 88mg; Carbohydrates: 63g; Fiber: 18g; Protein: 40g

Skillet Almond-Flour Halibut

GLUTEN-FREE, DAIRY-FREE, NIGHTSHADE-FREE

SERVES 4 **PREP TIME:** 5 minutes **COOK TIME:** 10 minutes

Fried fish is a staple in the American diet, but deep-fried foods promote inflammation in the body. This simple panfried halibut is the ideal substitute and offers the health benefits of good quality fish without too much oil. In this recipe, the aquafaba, or liquid from a can of chickpeas (or white beans), acts like an egg wash to help the flour mixture stick to the halibut. Serve with a side of Wilted Spinach with Chickpeas (page 123).

¼ cup almond flour

1 teaspoon dried basil

½ teaspoon sea salt

¼ teaspoon freshly ground black pepper

1 (15-ounce) can chickpeas, drained, liquid reserved

4 (6-ounce) halibut fillets

2 tablespoons coconut oil

1. In a medium bowl, stir together the almond flour, basil, salt, and pepper until well mixed.

2. Pour the reserved chickpea liquid (aquafaba) in another medium bowl.

3. Dunk each halibut fillet into the aquafaba and immediately transfer it to the almond flour mixture, coating both sides of the fillet, and setting aside.

4. In a large skillet over medium heat, heat the coconut oil.

5. Place the coated fillets in the skillet and cook for 4 minutes, turn, and cook for 4 minutes more, or until the halibut reaches an internal temperature of 145°F and flakes easily with a fork.

Ingredient tip: To use aquafaba as an egg substitute in baked recipes, use 3 tablespoons of aquafaba in place of 1 large egg.

Per Serving: Calories: 349; Total Fat: 14g; Saturated Fat: 7g;

Cholesterol: 83mg; Carbohydrates: 16g; Fiber: 5g; Protein: 38g

Broiled Halibut with Squash and Onions

GLUTEN-FREE, DAIRY-FREE, NIGHTSHADE-FREE
SERVES 4 **PREP TIME:** 10 minutes **COOK TIME:** 20 minutes

Sheet pan dinners are an excellent way to create a nutritious meal with minimal cleanup. This recipe features halibut, which is high in anti-inflammatory omega-3 fatty acids and also contains selenium, which can help lower inflammation in the body. Halibut is also a great source of magnesium, a mineral that's involved in hundreds of reactions in the body—and something most Americans lack in their diet.

2 large yellow squash, thinly sliced

2 large yellow onions, thinly sliced

3 tablespoons avocado oil, divided

1 teaspoon sea salt, divided

½ teaspoon freshly ground black pepper, divided

4 (6-ounce) halibut fillets

½ teaspoon dried thyme

1. Preheat the broiler to low. Line a sheet pan with parchment paper.

2. In a medium bowl, combine the squash and onions.

3. Add 2 tablespoons oil, ½ teaspoon salt, and ¼ teaspoon pepper and mix well. Place the squash mixture on one end of the prepared sheet pan.

4. Broil for 8 minutes.

5. Remove the pan from the oven. Place the halibut fillets on the sheet pan and brush with the remaining 1 tablespoon oil and sprinkle with the remaining ½ teaspoon salt, remaining ¼ teaspoon pepper, and thyme.

6. Broil for 10 minutes, or until the fish reaches an internal temperature of 145°F and flakes easily with a fork.

Ingredient tip: Choose wild-caught halibut over farmed to minimize toxins and contaminants.

Per Serving: Calories: 303; Total Fat: 13g; Saturated Fat: 2g;

Cholesterol: 83mg; Carbohydrates: 12g; Fiber: 3g; Protein: 34g

Baked Salmon with Fruit Salsa

DAIRY-FREE, GLUTEN-FREE
SERVES 4 **PREP TIME:** 10 minutes **COOK TIME:** 30 minutes

Eating fatty fish, salmon, at least twice a week is a great way to take advantage of anti-inflammatory omega-3 fatty acids. The colorful fruit salsa adds a tangy twist to this dish, while the pineapple, tomato, and bell peppers provide vitamin C for a healthy immune system.

4 (6-ounce) salmon fillets

2 tablespoons freshly squeezed lemon juice

1 teaspoon dried rosemary

½ teaspoon sea salt

¼ teaspoon freshly ground black pepper

⅓ cup water

¼ cup diced pineapple

½ medium red onion, diced

3 garlic cloves, minced

1 medium jalapeño pepper, diced

1 medium Roma tomato, diced

1 tablespoon honey

½ medium red bell pepper, diced

½ medium yellow bell pepper, diced

1 tablespoon dried basil

1. Preheat the oven to 350°F.

2. Place the salmon fillets in a shallow baking dish and season with the lemon juice, rosemary, salt, and pepper. Pour the water into the dish around the fillets.

3. Bake for 30 minutes, or until the salmon reaches an internal temperature of 145°F and flakes easily with a fork.

4. Meanwhile, in a medium bowl, stir together the pineapple, red onion, garlic, jalapeño, tomato, honey, red and yellow bell peppers, and basil. Cover the salsa mixture and refrigerate until the fish is cooked.

5. To serve, top each salmon fillet with an equal amount of fruit salad.

Ingredient tip: When choosing salmon, look for wild-caught Alaskan varieties to avoid high levels of contaminants. SeafoodWatch.org is a great resource for finding healthy seafood options.

Per Serving: Calories: 240; Total Fat: 7g; Saturated Fat: 2g; Cholesterol: 83mg; Carbohydrates: 11g; Fiber: 2g; Protein: 34g

Halibut and Dark Greens Skillet

GLUTEN-FREE, DAIRY-FREE, NIGHTSHADE-FREE

SERVES 4 PREP TIME: 10 minutes COOK TIME: 20 minutes

Swiss chard is a great source of vitamins A, C, and K, and it also contains magnesium, vitamin E and fiber. The nutrients in this super green—along with its polyphenol content—provide powerful antioxidant and anti-inflammatory benefits. When you pair the power of greens with the omega-3 fatty acids in the halibut, you get a recipe that's mighty for targeting inflammation.

¼ cup coconut oil

¾ cup gluten-free oat flour

2 shallots, minced

3 teaspoons dried parsley

1 tablespoon freshly squeezed lemon juice

1 teaspoon sea salt, divided

½ teaspoon freshly ground black pepper, divided

4 tablespoons avocado oil, divided

4 (6-ounce) halibut fillets

8 cups coarsely chopped rainbow Swiss chard

2 tablespoons water

1. Preheat the oven to 350°F.

2. In a small saucepan over medium heat, melt the coconut oil. Add the oat flour, half the minced shallots, parsley, lemon juice, ½ teaspoon salt, and ¼ teaspoon pepper and stir until combined. Remove from the heat.

3. Brush 1½ teaspoons avocado oil on each fillet and lay them on a plate.

4. Place an equal amount of the oat flour mixture (about 3 tablespoons) on top of each halibut fillet and press the mixture into the fillets.

5. In a cast-iron skillet over medium heat, heat the remaining 2 tablespoons avocado oil. Add the remaining shallots and the Swiss chard and sauté for 3 minutes, or until wilted.

6. Add the water, remaining ½ teaspoon salt, and remaining ¼ teaspoon pepper to the wilted Swiss chard and mix well.

7. Lay the halibut fillets on top of the Swiss chard and transfer the skillet to the oven.

8. Bake for 15 minutes, or until the halibut reaches an internal temperature of 145°F and flakes easily with a fork.

Variation tip: Instead of Swiss chard, use an equal amount of chopped red kale with the stems removed to add a slightly sweet, nutty flavor to this recipe.

Per Serving: Calories: 527; Total Fat: 31g; Saturated Fat: 14g; Cholesterol: 83mg; Carbohydrates: 25g; Fiber: 5g; Protein: 37g

Ginger Salmon with Macadamia Nuts

DAIRY-FREE, GLUTEN-FREE, NIGHTSHADE-FREE

SERVES 4 PREP TIME: 5 minutes COOK TIME: 15 minutes

In addition to the anti-inflammatory omega-3 fatty acids in salmon and gingerol in fresh ginger, this recipe also includes the health benefits of macadamia nuts. When you eat nuts, the bacteria in your gut ferment them to create short chain fatty acids that serve as fuel for the cells of your colon and help prevent inflammatory diseases. Nuts also help control blood sugar and triglyceride levels.

4 (6-ounce) salmon fillets

¼ teaspoon sea salt

1 tablespoon honey

1 tablespoon soy-free coconut aminos

1 tablespoon Dijon mustard

1 tablespoon minced peeled fresh ginger

½ cup raw macadamia nuts, chopped

1. Preheat the oven to 425°F. Line a baking sheet with parchment paper.

2. Place the salmon fillets on the prepared baking sheet and season with salt.

3. In a small bowl, stir together the honey, coconut aminos, mustard, and ginger. Using a pastry brush, gently brush each salmon fillet with the mustard mixture.

4. Sprinkle the filets with the macadamia nuts.

5. Bake for 15 minutes, or until the salmon reaches an internal temperature of 145°F and flakes easily with a fork.

Ingredient tip: Coconut aminos are a gluten-free and soy-free soy sauce substitute made from the fermented sap of the coconut palm tree. This condiment has a slightly sweet and salty flavor and can be found in grocery stores or online.

Per Serving: Calories: 321; Total Fat: 18g; Saturated Fat: 4g; Cholesterol: 83mg; Carbohydrates: 8g; Fiber: 1g; Protein: 34g

Sheet Pan Almond-Butter Salmon and Broccoli

DAIRY-FREE, GLUTEN-FREE, NIGHTSHADE-FREE

SERVES 4 PREP TIME: 10 minutes **COOK TIME:** 15 minutes

This recipe has it all! The almond butter adds a rich, nutty flavor to balance the more savory salmon, and it also offers healthy monounsaturated fats and protein. Along with inflammation-fighting omega-3 fats, this dish utilizes broccoli, which contains compounds such as sulforaphane, indole-3-carbinol, and quercetin to fight inflammation and cancer.

¼ cup soy-free coconut aminos

2 tablespoons almond butter

¼ cup apple cider vinegar with the mother

1 tablespoon honey

1 tablespoon extra-virgin olive oil

½ teaspoon garlic powder

½ teaspoon ground ginger

½ teaspoon sea salt

¼ teaspoon freshly ground black pepper

1 large head broccoli, chopped

4 (6-ounce) salmon fillets

1. Preheat the oven to 425°F. Line a large sheet pan with parchment paper.

2. In a small, lidded mason jar or salad dressing shaker, combine the coconut aminos, almond butter, vinegar, honey, oil, garlic powder, ginger, salt, and pepper. Seal the jar and shake well to combine.

3. In a medium bowl, combine the chopped broccoli and half the almond butter mixture. Mix well to coat.

4. Place the salmon fillets on one end of the prepared sheet pan and pour equal amounts of the remaining almond butter mixture over each fillet. Add the seasoned broccoli to the other end of the sheet pan.

5. Bake for 15 minutes, or until the salmon reaches an internal temperature of 145°F and flakes easily with a fork.

Ingredient tip: Many commercially prepared almond butters contain inflammatory oils and sugar. Look for varieties that only contain almonds and a little salt.

Per Serving: Calories: 361; Total Fat: 15g; Saturated Fat: 3g; Cholesterol: 83mg; Carbohydrates: 20g; Fiber: 5g; Protein: 39g

Honey-Baked Salmon

GLUTEN-FREE, DAIRY-FREE, NIGHTSHADE-FREE
SERVES 4 **PREP TIME:** 5 minutes **COOK TIME:** 15 minutes

Rich in omega-3 fatty acids, salmon helps quiet inflammation in the body. It's also a great source of protein to keep you feeling satisfied long after a meal is finished. The honey marinade adds a touch of sweetness, not to mention antioxidants. Serve with a side of Roasted Cauliflower "Steaks" (page 128) for a complete dinner.

½ cup honey

½ cup Dijon mustard

4 garlic cloves, minced

2 tablespoons freshly squeezed lemon juice

1 tablespoon extra-virgin olive oil

½ teaspoon dried basil

½ teaspoon onion powder

½ teaspoon ground cumin

½ teaspoon sea salt

¼ teaspoon freshly ground black pepper

1 (1-pound) salmon fillet

1. Preheat the oven to 400°F. Line a large baking sheet with parchment paper.

2. In a wide-mouthed, lidded mason jar, combine the honey, mustard, garlic, lemon juice, oil, basil, onion powder, cumin, salt, and pepper. Seal the jar and shake well to combine.

3. Place the salmon fillet in the center of the parchment paper and spread the honey mixture evenly over the fillet. Close the parchment by creating tight folds so the salmon is completely sealed in the parchment.

4. Bake for 15 minutes, or until the salmon reaches an internal temperature of 145°F and flakes easily with a fork.

5. Open the packet slowly to allow steam to escape and serve.

Ingredient tip: Marinating fish can enhance its flavor, but for a flaky fish like salmon, marinate it for no more than 30 minutes. To marinate the salmon in this recipe, put the salmon in a baking dish, pour the contents of the mason jar over the fish, cover, and refrigerate.

Per Serving: Calories: 327; Total Fat: 10g; Saturated Fat: 2g; Cholesterol: 55mg; Carbohydrates: 39g; Fiber: 1g; Protein: 24g

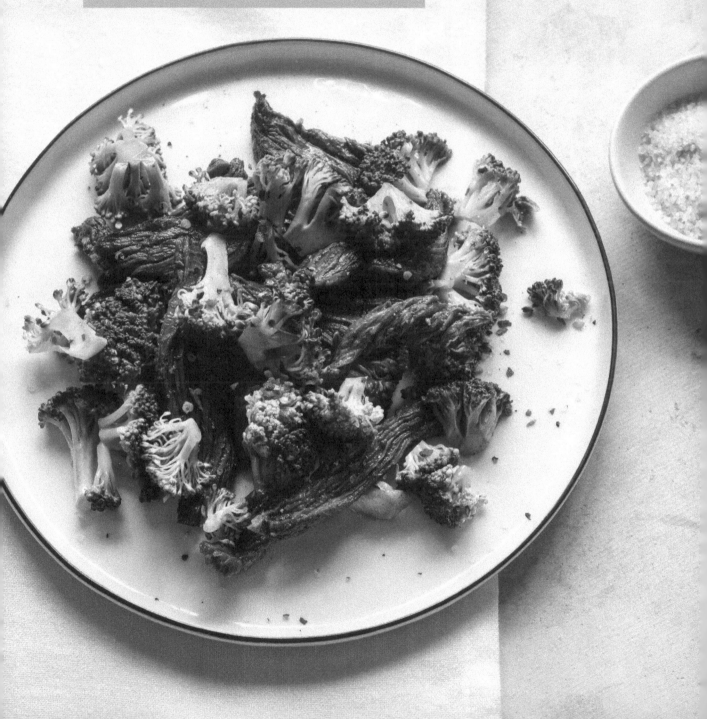

Healthy Beef and Broccoli Stir-Fry, page 106

7
POULTRY AND MEAT

Apple-Curry Turkey Salad

GLUTEN-FREE, DAIRY-FREE, NIGHTSHADE-FREE
SERVES 4 **PREP TIME:** 10 minutes **COOK TIME:** 10 minutes

This flavorful salad is packed with lean protein and paired with a tangy dressing and refreshing apples. Whole hemp seeds, the edible fruit of the *cannabis sativa* plant, provide a nutty flavor and add plenty of anti-inflammatory fats, healthy fibers, and an irresistible crunch to this dish.

2 tablespoons avocado oil

½ medium red onion, sliced

2 tablespoons freshly squeezed lemon juice

1 pound cooked turkey breast, cut into chunks

1 tablespoon nightshade-free curry powder (see page 68)

8 cups mixed greens, chopped

1 medium Gala apple, diced

¼ cup whole shelled hemp seeds

½ cup Simple Italian Salad Dressing (page 132)

1. In a medium skillet over medium heat, combine the oil and red onion and sauté for about 5 minutes, or until softened.

2. Add the lemon juice, turkey, and curry powder to the skillet and sauté for 5 minutes. Transfer to a large bowl and add the mixed greens, apple, hemp seeds, and dressing. Toss to coat and combine.

Ingredient tip: Choose organic turkey whenever possible, because conventionally raised turkeys are often kept in crowded conditions and not fed their natural diet. If you have trouble finding organic turkey, use 1 pound of organic chicken breast in this recipe.

Per Serving: Calories: 588; Total Fat: 42g; Saturated Fat: 6g; Cholesterol: 91mg; Carbohydrates: 16g; Fiber: 4g; Protein: 40g

Turkey and Cabbage Skillet

DAIRY-FREE, GLUTEN-FREE
SERVES 4 PREP TIME: 10 minutes COOK TIME: 35 minutes

This all-in-one recipe is perfect for dinner and it reheats well, making delicious leftovers. Cabbage, a powerful cruciferous vegetable, is an important source of vitamin C that supports a healthy immune system, and it reduces inflammation in the body. If you avoid nightshades, eliminate the diced tomatoes and instead add an extra onion.

2 tablespoons avocado oil

2 garlic cloves, chopped

1 medium yellow onion, chopped

1 pound ground turkey

1 small head green cabbage, coarsely chopped

1 (14.5-ounce) can diced tomatoes, with juices

1 teaspoon dried oregano

1 teaspoon dried basil

½ teaspoon dried thyme

½ teaspoon sea salt

¼ teaspoon freshly ground black pepper

1. In a large skillet or wok over medium heat, combine the oil and garlic and sauté for 3 minutes. Add the onion and sauté for 5 minutes.

2. Add the ground turkey and sauté for about 10 minutes, or until cooked through and no longer pink.

3. Add the cabbage, tomatoes with their juices, oregano, basil, thyme, salt, and pepper to the skillet and mix well. Cover the skillet and simmer over medium heat for 15 minutes, stirring frequently.

Variation tip: For a heartier meal, serve each portion over ½ cup of cooked quinoa.

Per Serving: Calories: 317; Total Fat: 17g; Saturated Fat: 3g;

Cholesterol: 84mg; Carbohydrates: 19g; Fiber: 6g; Protein: 25g

Creamy Avocado Chicken Salad

GLUTEN-FREE, DAIRY-FREE, NIGHTSHADE-FREE

SERVES 6 PREP TIME: 10 minutes **COOK TIME:** 15 minutes, plus 20 minutes to cool

This chicken salad skips the mayo and uses this fresh avocado dressing instead, which adds a dose of healthy monounsaturated fat and fiber to support a healthy gut microbiome. The crunchy walnuts help manage blood sugar and also have a prebiotic effect for healthy gut bacteria.

For the dressing

1½ ripe avocados, peeled, halved, and pitted

½ small cucumber

1 scallion, white and green parts, trimmed

1 tablespoon freshly squeezed lime juice

¼ cup extra-virgin olive oil

1 tablespoon apple cider vinegar with the mother

1 teaspoon honey

½ teaspoon dried dill weed

½ teaspoon dried basil

¼ teaspoon sea salt

¼ teaspoon freshly ground black pepper

For the chicken salad

2 tablespoons avocado oil

1 pound boneless, skinless chicken breasts, thinly sliced

2 celery stalks, diced

4 scallions, white and green parts, trimmed and chopped

½ cup red grapes, quartered

½ cup chopped walnuts

1. **To make the dressing:** In a small food processor, combine the avocados, cucumber, scallion, lime juice, olive oil, vinegar, honey, dill, basil, salt, and pepper. Process until smooth. Transfer the dressing to a large bowl.

2. **To make the chicken salad:** In a medium skillet over medium heat, heat the avocado oil. Add the chicken and sauté for 6 minutes. Flip the chicken breasts and sauté for 6 minutes more, or until the chicken reaches an internal temperature of 165°F.

3. Remove the cooked chicken from the heat and let cool for 20 minutes.

4. Place the chicken in a food processor and pulse until shredded, but do not overprocess.

5. Transfer the cooled chicken to the large bowl and add the dressing, celery, scallions, grapes, and walnuts. Toss to coat and combine.

Make it easier: Instead of using fresh chicken breasts, use 2 (12.5-ounce) cans of shredded chicken.

Per Serving: Calories: 349; Total Fat: 27g; Saturated Fat: 3g; Cholesterol: 53mg; Carbohydrates: 10g; Fiber: 4g; Protein: 19g

White Bean Turkey Chili

GLUTEN-FREE, DAIRY-FREE, NIGHTSHADE-FREE
SERVES 6 **PREP TIME:** 10 minutes **COOK TIME:** 35 minutes

Traditional chili often contains red meat and tomatoes, which can be inflammatory for some with autoimmune disease. This white bean version is just as tasty and provides a healthy dose of anti-inflammatory nutrients and fiber to support a healthy gut microbiome. Remember to look for organic, pasture-raised ground turkey.

1 tablespoon extra-virgin olive oil

1 medium yellow onion, chopped

2 celery stalks, chopped

2 medium carrots, diced

1 garlic clove, minced

1 teaspoon ground cumin

1 teaspoon ground coriander

1 teaspoon dried oregano

½ teaspoon sea salt

¼ teaspoon freshly ground black pepper

1 pound ground turkey

2 (15-ounce) cans cannellini beans, drained and rinsed

4 cups low-sodium vegetable broth

1. In a large Dutch oven over medium heat, combine the oil, onion, celery, and carrots. Sauté for about 8 minutes, or until the vegetables are softened.

2. Add the garlic, cumin, coriander, oregano, salt, and pepper and sauté for 3 minutes.

3. Add the ground turkey and sauté for about 4 minutes, stirring frequently.

4. Add the beans and broth. Increase the heat to high and bring the chili to a boil. Cover the pot and reduce the heat to medium. Cook for 20 minutes.

Batch cook tip: Although we often think of chili as a cold-weather food, this recipe is great all year long. It freezes well, so double the recipe and freeze the leftovers for up to 3 months for a quick meal option on hectic workdays.

Per Serving: Calories: 277; Total Fat: 10g; Saturated Fat: 2g; Cholesterol: 56mg; Carbohydrates: 26g; Fiber: 7g; Protein: 22g

Tangy Chicken with Quinoa

GLUTEN-FREE, DAIRY-FREE, NIGHTSHADE-FREE

SERVES 4 **PREP TIME:** 10 minutes **COOK TIME:** 20 minutes

In addition to the fiber and anti-inflammatory benefits of quinoa and greens, this recipe includes pepitas for a satisfying crunch. Pepitas are pumpkin seeds without the shell and are a great source of magnesium, which is involved in hundreds of reactions in the body.

2 cups water

1 cup red quinoa, rinsed

¼ cup balsamic vinegar

1 tablespoon freshly squeezed lime juice

½ teaspoon sea salt

¼ teaspoon freshly ground black pepper

⅓ cup extra-virgin olive oil

½ teaspoon dried dill weed

2 (12.5-ounce) cans shredded chicken breast, drained

1 cup fresh blueberries, halved

½ cup raw pepitas (shelled pumpkin seeds)

8 cups mixed greens

4 scallions, white and green part, trimmed and chopped

4 tablespoons whole shelled hemp seeds

1. In a small saucepan over high heat, combine the water and quinoa. Bring to a boil, cover the pan, and reduce the heat to low. Simmer for 15 minutes, until the quinoa absorbs the water. Remove the pan from the heat, leave covered, and let sit for 5 minutes.

2. Meanwhile, in a small bowl, whisk the vinegar, lime juice, salt, pepper, oil, and dill until combined.

3. In a large bowl, combine the cooked quinoa and half the dressing. Mix well to coat and combine.

4. Add the chicken, blueberries, pepitas, mixed greens, scallions, and remaining dressing and toss well to coat and combine.

5. Sprinkle each serving with 1 tablespoon hemp seeds.

Ingredient tip: You can substitute 2¾ cups of shredded baked chicken breast or shredded rotisserie chicken.

Per Serving: Calories: 657; Total Fat: 35g; Saturated Fat: 4g;
Cholesterol: 105mg; Carbohydrates: 46g; Fiber: 8g; Protein: 43g

Garlic Chicken and Cauliflower Rice

DAIRY-FREE, GLUTEN-FREE, NIGHTSHADE-FREE
SERVES 3 PREP TIME: 10 minutes **COOK TIME:** 20 minutes

This recipe is a great way to enjoy a variety of colorful vegetables while boosting overall nutrient and fiber intake. The real star of the show, however, is the mighty garlic, whose sulfur compounds help reduce inflammation and act as powerful antioxidants.

2 tablespoons avocado oil, divided

4 garlic cloves, minced

1 large red onion, cut into medium chunks

1 pound boneless, skinless chicken breasts, cut into 1-inch chunks

2 medium carrots, diced

1 medium head broccoli, cut into 1-inch chunks

3 tablespoons water

¾ cup low-sodium vegetable broth

½ cup soy-free coconut aminos

1 tablespoon coconut flour

1 tablespoon freshly squeezed lime juice

1 tablespoon minced peeled fresh ginger

1 teaspoon coconut sugar

½ teaspoon garlic powder

½ teaspoon sea salt

¼ teaspoon freshly ground black pepper

3 cups frozen riced cauliflower

1. In a large wok over medium heat, heat 1 tablespoon oil. Add the garlic and red onion and sauté for 3 minutes.

2. Add the chicken, carrots, broccoli, and water and sauté for 10 minutes, or until the vegetables are softened.

3. Meanwhile, in a small, lidded mason jar, combine the broth, coconut aminos, coconut flour, lime juice, ginger, coconut sugar, garlic powder, salt, and pepper. Seal the jar and shake well to combine.

4. To the wok, add the riced cauliflower and the remaining 1 tablespoon oil.

5. Add the broth mixture to the chicken mixture and stir well. Cover the wok and cook over medium heat for 5 minutes, or until heated through.

Per Serving: Calories: 461; Total Fat: 15g; Saturated Fat: 2g;

Cholesterol: 107mg; Carbohydrates: 42g; Fiber: 12g; Protein: 43g

Turmeric Chicken and Brown Rice

GLUTEN-FREE, DAIRY-FREE

SERVES 4 PREP TIME: 20 minutes **COOK TIME:** 35 minutes

This nourishing rice dish takes full advantage of anti-inflammatory spices such as turmeric, ginger, and cumin. It also calls for coriander to support a healthy immune system and cinnamon to reduce inflammation and improve blood sugar control. Cooking and cooling brown rice increases the amount of resistant starch for even more health benefits.

1 tablespoon coconut oil

2 garlic cloves, minced

1 medium yellow onion, chopped

1 medium carrot, shredded

1 medium red bell pepper, chopped

1 small zucchini, sliced

2 cups low-sodium chicken broth

⅔ cup raw brown rice

½ cup water

1 tablespoon ground turmeric

½ teaspoon ground ginger

½ teaspoon ground cumin

½ teaspoon ground coriander

½ teaspoon ground cinnamon

¼ teaspoon sea salt

¼ teaspoon freshly ground black pepper

1 pound boneless, skinless chicken breasts, cut into small chunks

1. In a Dutch oven over medium-high heat, combine the coconut oil, garlic, and onion and sauté for 4 minutes.

2. Add the carrot, bell pepper, and zucchini and sauté for 6 minutes, or until the vegetables are softened.

3. Add the broth, brown rice, and water and bring the mixture to a boil.

4. Stir in the turmeric, ginger, cumin, coriander, cinnamon, salt, and pepper.

5. Add the chicken to the mixture. Reduce the heat to medium-low and cook for 20 minutes, or until the chicken reaches an internal temperature of 165°F.

Substitution tip: If you avoid nightshades, omit the red bell pepper and add 1 medium yellow squash, sliced, instead.

Per Serving: Calories: 321; Total Fat: 8g; Saturated Fat: 4g; Cholesterol: 80mg;

Carbohydrates: 34g; Fiber: 4g; Protein: 29g

Pesto Chicken "Pasta"

GLUTEN-FREE, DAIRY-FREE, NIGHTSHADE-FREE
SERVES 4 **PREP TIME:** 10 minutes **COOK TIME:** 45 minutes

Traditional pesto recipes often include dairy. With this dairy-free version, you can enjoy all the vibrant flavors of pesto and the anti-inflammatory goodness of extra-virgin olive oil. The garlic, walnuts, and spinach provide fuel to keep the gut microbiome in balance. Spaghetti squash, which is full of antioxidants and fiber, is a great lower-calorie, lower-carbohydrate alternative to traditional pasta.

3 tablespoons avocado oil, divided

1 large spaghetti squash, halved and seeded

2 garlic cloves, minced, plus 2 whole garlic cloves, peeled

1 pound boneless, skinless chicken breasts, cut into chunks

2 cups fresh spinach

½ cup raw walnuts

¼ teaspoon sea salt

¼ teaspoon freshly ground black pepper

½ cup extra-virgin olive oil

1. Preheat the oven to 400°F. Line a baking sheet with parchment paper.

2. Drizzle 2 tablespoons avocado oil over the flesh of both spaghetti squash halves and place them on the prepared baking sheet, flesh-side down.

3. Bake for 45 minutes, or until tender.

4. Meanwhile, in a large skillet over medium heat, heat the remaining 1 tablespoon avocado oil. Add the minced garlic and sauté for 2 minutes.

5. Add the chicken and sauté for about 10 minutes, or until the chicken is golden brown and reaches an internal temperature of 165°F.

6. In a food processor, combine the spinach, walnuts, whole garlic cloves, salt, pepper, and olive oil. Process for about 45 seconds, or until smooth.

7. When the spaghetti squash is done, remove it from the oven and, using a fork, scrape the flesh into strands. Each half provides 2 servings of spaghetti squash.

8. To assemble, place one-fourth of the spaghetti squash on each plate, layer it with one-fourth of the chicken, and top each serving with 2 tablespoons spinach pesto.

Ingredient tip: The pesto recipe makes about 2½ cups. Refrigerate the leftovers in an airtight container for up to 3 days. Use it as a drizzle over roasted vegetables or as a dip for vegetable sticks.

Per Serving: Calories: 585; Total Fat: 47g; Saturated Fat: 6g; Cholesterol: 80mg; Carbohydrates: 16g; Fiber: 4g; Protein: 29g

Spice-Rubbed Chicken Breast

GLUTEN-FREE, DAIRY-FREE, NIGHTSHADE-FREE

SERVES 4 **PREP TIME:** 10 minutes **COOK TIME:** 20 minutes

This flavorful dish harnesses the deep flavors and anti-inflammatory benefits of turmeric, cumin, curry, cinnamon, and cloves to jazz up plain chicken breast. Cloves also contain eugenol, a potent antioxidant shown to have anti-cancer properties and improve liver health. Serve it with Simple Roasted Vegetables (page 126) and Carrot Salad with Spicy Greens (page 124).

2 teaspoons freshly ground black pepper

1½ teaspoons ground cumin

1½ teaspoons nightshade-free curry powder (see page 68)

½ teaspoon ground turmeric

½ teaspoon ground cinnamon

¼ teaspoon ground cloves

1 pound boneless, skinless chicken breasts (4 breasts)

½ teaspoon sea salt

2 tablespoons avocado oil

1. In a small bowl, stir together the pepper, cumin, curry powder, turmeric, cinnamon, and cloves until combined. Set aside.

2. Place the chicken breasts on a plate and, using your hands, rub each with a sprinkle of salt on both sides. Then, rub the spice mixture onto each chicken breast, patting the breasts to coat.

3. In a large skillet over medium heat, heat the oil. Add the chicken. Cook for 8 minutes per side, or until the chicken reaches an internal temperature of 165°F.

Batch cook tip: I like using this chicken in the Pesto Chicken "Pasta" (page 100) and Creamy Avocado Chicken Salad (page 94) recipes. Double this recipe and refrigerate the chicken in an airtight container for up to 5 days to use with either of those recipes.

Per Serving: Calories: 201; Total Fat: 10g; Saturated Fat: 1g;

Cholesterol: 80mg; Carbohydrates: 2g; Fiber: 1g; Protein: 25g

Roasted Chicken Thighs

GLUTEN-FREE, DAIRY-FREE, NIGHTSHADE-FREE
SERVES 4 **PREP TIME:** 5 minutes, plus 1 hour to marinate **COOK TIME:** 30 minutes

Chicken thighs are a great source of protein, while also providing important B vitamins and minerals including iron, selenium, and zinc. Chicken thighs are higher in fat than skinless chicken breasts, but that extra fat adds flavor and enhances satiety. To complete the meal, pair this dish with Baked Sweet Potato Fries (page 131) and Garlic Brussels Sprouts (page 129).

½ cup extra-virgin olive oil

2 tablespoons balsamic vinegar

1 tablespoon Dijon mustard

1 tablespoon honey

½ teaspoon kosher salt

¼ teaspoon freshly ground black pepper

4 (4-ounce) boneless, skinless chicken thighs

1. Preheat the oven to 375°F. Line a baking sheet with parchment paper.

2. In a medium bowl, whisk the oil, vinegar, mustard, honey, salt, and pepper until blended. Add the chicken to the bowl and toss it with the dressing. Cover and refrigerate to marinate for 1 hour, or up to overnight.

3. Spread the marinated chicken on the prepared baking sheet.

4. Roast for 20 minutes. Flip the chicken and roast for 10 minutes more, or until the internal temperature reaches 165°F.

Make it easier: Prepare these chicken thighs the night before you plan to serve them. Then, cover and let them marinate overnight in the refrigerator.

Per Serving: Calories: 397; Total Fat: 34g; Saturated Fat: 4g;
Cholesterol: 91mg; Carbohydrates: 6g; Fiber: <1g; Protein: 18g

Sheet Pan Mediterranean Chicken

GLUTEN-FREE, DAIRY-FREE, NIGHTSHADE-FREE

SERVES 4 **PREP TIME:** 10 minutes **COOK TIME:** 45 minutes

This all-in-one sheet pan dinner includes a lean protein, healthy carbohydrate, and savory seasoned vegetables. Sweet potatoes offer important cancer-fighting and anti-inflammatory benefits and can help manage blood sugar.

¼ cup extra-virgin olive oil

2 tablespoons freshly squeezed lemon juice

4 garlic cloves, minced

1 tablespoon dried oregano

1½ teaspoons dried basil

¾ teaspoon sea salt

¼ teaspoon freshly ground black pepper

1 pound boneless, skinless breasts (4 breasts)

2 medium sweet potatoes, cut into small chunks

1 large red onion, cut into chunks

1 large zucchini, cut into chunks

1 large yellow squash, cut into chunks

1. Preheat the oven to 350°F. Line a large sheet pan with parchment paper.

2. In a small bowl, whisk the oil, lemon juice, garlic, oregano, basil, salt, and pepper until well mixed.

3. Place the chicken breasts on one end of the prepared sheet pan. Using a pastry brush, coat each chicken breast with the oil mixture, reserving the remaining oil.

4. In a medium bowl, combine the sweet potatoes, red onion, zucchini, squash, and the remaining oil mixture and mix well to coat and combine. Add the vegetables to the sheet pan with the chicken.

5. Bake for 30 minutes. Turn the chicken over and stir the vegetables around. Bake for 15 minutes more, or until the chicken reaches an internal temperature of 165°F.

Per Serving: Calories: 357; Total Fat: 17g; Saturated Fat: 3g;

Cholesterol: 80mg; Carbohydrates: 24g; Fiber: 5g; Protein: 29g

Hearty Chicken Stew

GLUTEN-FREE, DAIRY-FREE, NIGHTSHADE-FREE

SERVES 6 **PREP TIME:** 10 minutes **COOK TIME:** 50 minutes

This all-in-one stew combines the anti-inflammatory benefits of coriander, cumin, and ginger with sweet potatoes, which are full of fiber for a healthy gut. The coconut cream creates a creamy texture without affecting the flavor and is a good source of medium-chain triglycerides, which are easily absorbed by the body for energy, and can improve gut health by nourishing the gastrointestinal lining.

3 (4-ounce) boneless, skinless chicken breasts, cut into chunks

½ teaspoon sea salt

¼ teaspoon freshly ground black pepper

3 tablespoons extra-virgin olive oil, divided

1 medium red onion, chopped

1 tablespoon grated peeled fresh ginger

4 garlic cloves, minced

1 tablespoon ground cumin

2 teaspoons ground coriander

4 cups low-sodium chicken broth

½ cup coconut cream

3 small sweet potatoes, diced

1. In a medium bowl, stir together the chicken chunks, salt, and pepper.

2. In a Dutch oven over medium heat, heat 2 tablespoons oil. Add the chicken and sauté for 5 minutes, stirring frequently, until browned.

3. Add the remaining 1 tablespoon oil, red onion, ginger, and garlic to the pot and sauté for 5 minutes, or until softened.

4. Stir in the cumin and coriander and sauté for 3 minutes.

5. Add the broth, coconut cream, and sweet potatoes. Increase the heat to high and bring the stew to a boil. Reduce the heat to medium-low and simmer for 35 minutes, or until the flavors are incorporated.

Batch cook tip: This stew freezes well. Double it and freeze in an airtight container for up to 3 months for a quick, hearty meal when life gets hectic.

Per Serving: Calories: 236; Total Fat: 12g; Saturated Fat: 4g; Cholesterol: 40mg; Carbohydrates: 18g; Fiber: 2g; Protein: 14g

Healthy Beef and Broccoli Stir-Fry

GLUTEN-FREE, DAIRY-FREE, NIGHTSHADE-FREE

SERVES 4 **PREP TIME:** 10 minutes **COOK TIME:** 20 minutes

When I went soy-free, I thought I would have to give up stir-fry. Not with this stir-fry recipe, which offers a flavorful, satisfying soy-free alternative thanks to the use of coconut aminos and fresh ginger. It's also a delicious way to enjoy the prebiotic benefit of leeks and health-promoting broccoli. This dish reheats very well, so it's a great leftover option for lunch.

1 tablespoon avocado oil

1 pound flank steak, cut into chunks

½ teaspoon sea salt

¼ teaspoon freshly ground black pepper

4 cups fresh or frozen broccoli

1 large leek, trimmed, cleaned well, and cut into rings

1 large carrot, sliced

¾ cup soy-free coconut aminos

1 garlic clove, minced

1 tablespoon minced peeled fresh ginger

1 tablespoon almond flour

1 tablespoon honey

1. In a large skillet or wok over medium-high heat, heat the oil. Add the steak and season with the salt and pepper. Cook for 8 minutes, stirring frequently.

2. Add the broccoli, leek, and carrot to the skillet. Cover the skillet and cook for about 5 minutes, or until the vegetables are tender and the steak is cooked through or reaches an internal temperature of 145°F.

3. While the steak and vegetables cook, in a small, lidded mason jar, combine the coconut aminos, garlic, ginger, almond flour, and honey. Seal the jar and shake well to combine. Add the sauce to the steak and vegetables and mix well. Cook, uncovered, stirring frequently, for 5 minutes.

Substitution tip: If you tolerate nightshades, add 1 large orange bell pepper, cut into strips, to add even more vibrant color and flavor.

Per Serving: Calories: 358; Total Fat: 15g; Saturated Fat: 5g;

Cholesterol: 55mg; Carbohydrates: 26g; Fiber: 4g; Protein: 28g

Rosemary Steak and Spicy Greens

GLUTEN-FREE, DAIRY-FREE, NIGHTSHADE-FREE

SERVES 4 **PREP TIME:** 10 minutes, plus 2 hours to marinate **COOK TIME:** 15 minutes

The psoriasis meal plan in this book offers limited amounts of red meat because conventionally raised red meat can create inflammation in the body. When choosing beef, look for organic, grass-fed, local options if possible, which have higher amounts of anti-inflammatory omega-3 fatty acids and conjugated linoleic acid (CLA), a powerful antioxidant. This recipe also calls for immune-boosting rosemary and spicy, fiber-rich arugula.

¼ cup extra-virgin olive oil

1 tablespoon apple cider vinegar with the mother

1 garlic clove, minced

2 teaspoons dried rosemary

½ teaspoon sea salt

½ teaspoon freshly ground black pepper

1 (1-pound) sirloin steak

8 cups arugula

½ cup Simple Italian Salad Dressing (page 132)

1. In a small bowl, whisk the oil, vinegar, garlic, rosemary, salt, and pepper to blend.

2. Place the steak in a glass dish with a lid and pour the marinade over the steak. Cover the dish and refrigerate the steak for at least 2 hours, or up to overnight.

3. In a large skillet over medium heat, cook the steak for 8 minutes. Flip the steak and cook for 8 minutes more, or until it reaches an internal temperature of 145°F. Remove from the heat, let rest for 10 minutes, then slice the steak.

4. To serve, place 2 cups arugula on each of four plates. Top each serving with one-fourth of the steak and drizzle with 2 tablespoons dressing.

Make it easier: Prepare the marinade the day before, pour it over the steaks, cover, and let marinate in the refrigerator overnight.

Per Serving: Calories: 623; Total Fat: 57g; Saturated Fat: 12g;
Cholesterol: 90mg; Carbohydrates: 3g; Fiber: 1g; Protein: 24g

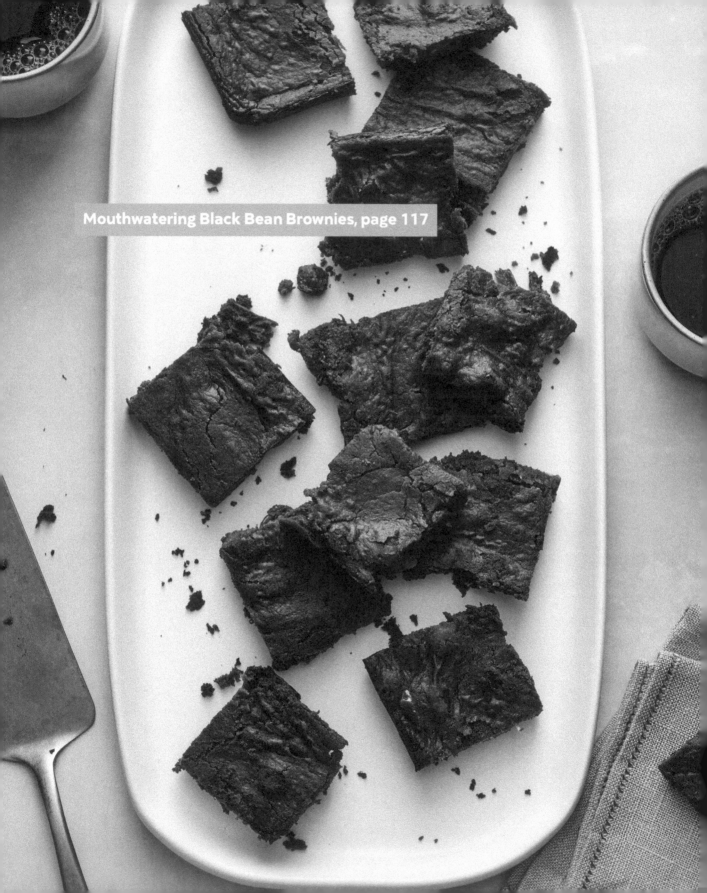

Mouthwatering Black Bean Brownies, page 117

8
DESSERTS

Gluten-Free Apple Crisp

DAIRY-FREE, GLUTEN-FREE, NIGHTSHADE-FREE, VEGAN

SERVES 6 PREP TIME: 15 minutes COOK TIME: 45 minutes

My mom makes wonderful apple dumplings with the most perfect crumbly topping. This recipe is my version— without the inflammatory ingredients. Apples can help decrease inflammation and improve blood lipid and blood sugar levels in the body. Choose certified gluten-free oats to avoid cross-contamination.

For the apple crisp

1 teaspoon coconut oil, melted

5 medium Gala apples, chopped into chunks

¼ cup pure maple syrup

1 tablespoon freshly squeezed lemon juice

1 teaspoon vanilla extract

1 teaspoon ground cinnamon

1 tablespoon tapioca flour

1 tablespoon coconut sugar

For the topping

½ cup gluten-free oat flour

¼ cup tapioca flour

1 tablespoon coconut sugar

½ cup chopped pecans

3 tablespoons pure maple syrup

3 tablespoons coconut oil

1 teaspoon baking powder

¼ teaspoon sea salt

1. Preheat the oven to 350°F. Coat a 9-inch pie pan with the melted coconut oil.

2. **To make the apple crisp:** In a large bowl, stir together the apples, maple syrup, lemon juice, vanilla, cinnamon, and tapioca flour until well combined. Transfer the apple mixture to the prepared pie pan and sprinkle the coconut sugar evenly over the top.

3. **To make the topping:** In a food processor, combine the oat flour, tapioca flour, coconut sugar, pecans, maple syrup, coconut oil, baking powder, and salt. Pulse until all ingredients are incorporated. Sprinkle the topping over the apple mixture in an even layer (the topping will be somewhat chunky).

4. Bake for 45 minutes, until the topping is golden brown.

Per Serving: Calories: 346; Total Fat: 15g; Saturated Fat: 7g; Cholesterol: 0mg; Carbohydrates: 55g; Fiber: 63g; Protein: 3g

Cookie Dough Bars

DAIRY-FREE, GLUTEN-FREE, NIGHTSHADE-FREE, VEGETARIAN

SERVES 12 **PREP TIME:** 15 minutes, plus 1 hour to chill

These rich Cookie Dough Bars are a great dessert and also a wonderful pre- or post-workout snack. Along with healthy fat and protein, they contain cacao. Cacao nibs and cacao powder are known for the health-promoting benefits of their flavonols, which act as antioxidants but may also decrease obesity-related inflammation. As well, cacao flavonols boost the numbers of health-promoting bacteria while decreasing less beneficial microbes.

1½ cups cashew butter

½ cup mashed peeled, cooked sweet potato

2¼ cups almond flour

3 tablespoons coconut milk

⅓ cup cacao nibs

¼ cup honey

1½ tablespoons cacao powder

2 tablespoons pecan butter

1. Line an 8-by8-inch freezer-safe dish with parchment paper.

2. In a food processor, combine the cashew butter, mashed sweet potato, almond flour, coconut milk, cacao nibs, and honey. Blend until smooth. Transfer about three-fourths of the cashew butter mixture to the prepared dish, spreading it into an even layer.

3. Add the cacao powder and pecan butter to the remaining cashew butter mixture in the food processor and process until incorporated. Spread this mixture over the cashew mixture in the dish and smooth the top.

4. Cover the dish and freeze for at least 1 hour.

5. Cut into 12 servings and keep refrigerated in an airtight container for up to 7 days.

Ingredient tip: Cacao nibs and cacao powder can be found in most grocery and health food stores or online. While cacao powder and cocoa powder are similar, cacao powder is processed at lower temperatures and retains more of the nutritional benefits of cacao.

Per Serving: Calories: 384; Total Fat: 30g; Saturated Fat: 6g; Cholesterol: 0mg; Carbohydrates: 23g; Fiber: 4g; Protein: 11g

Chunky Chocolate Banana Bread

DAIRY-FREE, GLUTEN-FREE, NIGHTSHADE-FREE, VEGAN

SERVES 12 **PREP TIME:** 15 minutes **COOK TIME:** 40 minutes

Banana bread is a wonderful comfort food, but it usually includes butter, sugar, and eggs. This version is more wholesome and just as delicious. The flaxseed and banana provide fiber to fuel the gut microbiome, and the flavonols in dark chocolate also deliver benefits to the gut microbiome. Bananas are also a great source of potassium, which is important for controlling blood pressure. If you've only got unripe bananas, go ahead and use them—they are an excellent source of resistant starch for balancing the gut microbiome!

2 tablespoons whole-milled flaxseed

6 tablespoons water

4 small bananas, mashed (about 2½ cups)

½ cup unsweetened applesauce

½ cup almond butter

¼ cup coconut oil, melted

½ cup coconut flour

½ teaspoon ground cinnamon

1 teaspoon baking powder

1 teaspoon baking soda

1 teaspoon vanilla extract

¼ teaspoon sea salt

½ cup dairy-free vegan dark chocolate chips

1. To create the flax "eggs," in a small bowl, stir together the flaxseed and water and let sit for 10 minutes to thicken.

2. Preheat the oven to 350°F. Line an 8-by-8-inch baking pan or 9-by-5-inch loaf pan with parchment paper.

3. In a large bowl, stir together the bananas, applesauce, almond butter, melted coconut oil, and flax "eggs" until well mixed.

4. Add the coconut flour, cinnamon, baking powder, baking soda, vanilla, and salt to the banana mixture and mix well.

5. Fold in the chocolate chips. Transfer the batter to the prepared baking pan.

6. Bake for 40 minutes, until golden brown and a toothpick inserted into the center comes out clean. Remove from the oven and let completely cool before slicing.

Ingredient tip: Allergen-free chocolate chips are available in most grocery or health food stores. To make your own, in a medium bowl, stir together ½ cup of melted coconut oil, ½ cup of cacao powder, 2 tablespoons of pure maple syrup, ¼ teaspoon of sea salt, and 1 teaspoon of vanilla extract and pour into a shallow pan. Cover and chill in the refrigerator for 2 hours, until hard. Break the chocolate into chunks and use ½ cup of chunks in place of the dark chocolate chips.

Per Serving: Calories: 214; Total Fat: 15g; Saturated Fat: 7g; Cholesterol: <1mg; Carbohydrates: 18g; Fiber: 5g; Protein: 4g

Walnut Blondie Brownies

DAIRY-FREE, GLUTEN-FREE, NIGHTSHADE-FREE, VEGETARIAN
SERVES 9 PREP TIME: 10 minutes COOK TIME: 25 minutes

Using beans to make brownies may sound like a stretch, but these wholesome brownies taste fantastic, and I promise you won't taste the beans at all! And you'll never know there is no white chocolate, thanks to the creamy texture from the almond butter and the perfect touch of sweetness from the honey. It's best to store these brownies in the refrigerator for up to 5 days.

1½ cups canned great northern beans, drained and rinsed

½ teaspoon baking powder

¼ teaspoon sea salt

½ cup honey

2 teaspoons vanilla extract

½ cup certified gluten-free rolled oats

¼ cup coconut oil, melted

2 tablespoons almond butter

½ cup chopped walnuts

1. Preheat the oven to 350°F. Line an 8-by-8-inch baking dish with parchment paper.

2. In a food processor, combine the beans, baking powder, salt, honey, vanilla, oats, melted coconut oil, and almond butter. Process until smooth. Transfer the mixture to a medium bowl.

3. Fold in the walnuts. Spread the mixture into the prepared baking dish.

4. Bake for 25 minutes, or until golden brown. Cool completely before cutting into 9 squares.

Substitution tip: An equal amount of chickpeas can be substituted for the great northern beans.

Per Serving: Calories: 234; Total Fat: 13g; Saturated Fat: 6g; Cholesterol: 0mg; Carbohydrates: 28g; Fiber: 3g; Protein: 5g

Blueberry Chia Pudding

DAIRY-FREE, GLUTEN-FREE, NIGHTSHADE-FREE, VEGAN
SERVES 4 PREP TIME: 10 minutes, plus overnight to chill

Chia seeds are an amazing source of gut-friendly fiber, and they are packed with antioxidants and anti-inflammatory benefits. Chia seeds are a great source of plant-based protein for vegans and vegetarians, too. The blueberries add even more antioxidants, which are important for brain, heart, and metabolic health. This refreshing dessert also works well as a simple breakfast pudding.

1¼ cups Creamy Cashew Milk (page 133) or other nut milk, such as almond or coconut

6 tablespoons chia seeds

½ cup frozen blueberries

2 tablespoons pure maple syrup

½ teaspoon vanilla extract

1 teaspoon ground cinnamon

1. In a blender, combine the cashew milk, chia seeds, blueberries, maple syrup, vanilla, and cinnamon. Blend until combined.

2. Divide the pudding among four small mason jars (about ½ cup in each) and chill overnight in the refrigerator.

Variation tip: For a more decadent chocolate version, add ¼ cup of cacao powder with the other ingredients.

Per Serving: Calories: 192; Total Fat: 10g; Saturated Fat: 1g; Cholesterol: 0mg; Carbohydrates: 22g; Fiber: 9g; Protein: 5g

Vanilla Protein Bites

DAIRY-FREE, GLUTEN-FREE, NIGHTSHADE-FREE, VEGAN
SERVES 12 PREP TIME: 10 minutes

These protein bites are a delicious pre- or post-workout snack, and they're also great as an after-dinner treat. They contain Medjool dates, which have been shown to lower triglyceride levels and decrease oxidative stress in the body without increasing blood sugar. The cashews and macadamia nuts add a healthy dose of prebiotics to keep the gut microbiome healthy and reduce chronic inflammation.

⅔ cup raw cashews

⅔ cup raw
macadamia nuts

1 scoop vegan vanilla
protein powder

½ teaspoon sea salt

1 cup Medjool dates,
pitted and halved

1 tablespoon pure
maple syrup

1 tablespoon coconut
oil, melted

1. In a food processor, combine the cashews and macadamia nuts and pulse for about 20 seconds, until finely ground.

2. Add the protein powder and salt and pulse for about 15 seconds, until combined.

3. Add the dates, maple syrup, and melted coconut oil and process for 45 seconds to 1 minute, until the ingredients are incorporated and the mixture is sticky.

4. Using your hands, form the mixture into 12 balls and refrigerate in an airtight container for up to 7 days.

Batch cook tip: To make a chocolate version, use a vegan chocolate protein powder, or add 2 tablespoons of cacao powder with the vanilla protein powder.

Per Serving: Calories: 175; Total Fat: 10g; Saturated Fat: 2g; Cholesterol: 0mg; Carbohydrates: 21g; Fiber: 3g; Protein: 4g

Mouthwatering Black Bean Brownies

DAIRY-FREE, GLUTEN-FREE, NIGHTSHADE-FREE, VEGAN

SERVES 16   **PREP TIME:** 15 minutes   **COOK TIME:** 30 minutes

These decadent brownies will make you wonder why you've not used black beans in dessert recipes before. Black beans are a great source of plant-based protein, and they offer resistant starch and fiber to keep the gut microbiome in balance. They also contain phytonutrients that act as antioxidants in the body. When you consider you also get antioxidant flavonols from the cacao powder, these brownies make the perfect anti-inflammatory treat.

1 tablespoon whole-milled flaxseed

3 tablespoons water

1 (15-ounce) can black beans, drained and rinsed

½ cup coconut sugar

¼ cup cacao powder

¼ cup canned pure pumpkin

3 tablespoons coconut oil (solid, not melted)

½ teaspoon sea salt

½ teaspoon baking powder

½ cup dairy-free vegan dark chocolate chips (optional)

1. Preheat the oven to 350°F. Line a 9-by-13-inch baking dish with parchment paper.

2. In a small bowl, make a flax "egg" by stirring together the flaxseed and water. Let sit for 10 minutes to thicken.

3. In a food processer, combine the flax "egg," black beans, coconut sugar, cacao powder, pumpkin, coconut oil, salt, and baking powder. Process until smooth. Transfer the mixture to a large bowl.

4. Fold in the chocolate chips (if using). Spread the batter in the prepared baking dish.

5. Bake for 30 minutes. Let completely cool before cutting into 16 squares.

Ingredient tip: Made from the sap of the coconut palm plant, coconut sugar is available in most grocery stores. Although it does offer some nutrients and has a slightly lower effect on blood sugar than other more conventional sugars, it is still an added sugar and should be used in moderation.

Per Serving: Calories: 83; Total Fat: 3g; Saturated Fat: 2g; Cholesterol: 0mg; Carbohydrates: 12g; Fiber: 3g; Protein: 2g

Cranberry Cookies

DAIRY-FREE, GLUTEN-FREE, NIGHTSHADE-FREE, VEGAN

SERVES 12 **PREP TIME:** 20 minutes **COOK TIME:** 10 minutes

Giving up gluten and eggs doesn't have to mean giving up cookies. These Cranberry Cookies make a great after-dinner treat or a delicious breakfast. Fiber-rich oats contain a polyphenol called avenanthramide, which helps lower inflammation.

1 tablespoon whole-milled flaxseed

3 tablespoons water

¼ cup coconut oil (solid, not melted)

¼ cup coconut sugar

2 tablespoons pure maple syrup

1 teaspoon vanilla extract

2 cups certified gluten-free rolled oats

½ teaspoon baking soda

¼ teaspoon sea salt

⅓ cup chopped pecans

⅓ cup dried cranberries

1. Preheat the oven to 350°F. Line a baking sheet with parchment paper.

2. In a small bowl, stir together the flaxseed and water. Let sit for 10 minutes to thicken.

3. In a medium bowl and using a handheld mixer, or in the bowl of a stand mixer fitted with the paddle attachment, combine the flax mixture, coconut oil, coconut sugar, maple syrup, and vanilla. Mix on medium speed until incorporated.

4. Add the oats, baking soda, and salt and mix on medium speed until incorporated.

5. Fold in the pecans and cranberries.

6. Using your hands, form 1½ tablespoons of cookie dough into a ball and place on the prepared baking sheet. Repeat with the remaining dough to create 12 balls. Gently press each cookie ball with the back of a fork to flatten slightly.

7. Bake for 8 minutes, or until golden brown. Remove from the oven and, again, press the cookies with the back of the fork to flatten. Let cool completely.

8. Refrigerate in an airtight container for up to 5 days.

Per Serving: Calories: 153; Total Fat: 8g; Saturated Fat: 4g; Cholesterol: 0mg;

Carbohydrates: 20g; Fiber: 2g; Protein: 2g

Creamy Cashew Milk Ice Cream

DAIRY-FREE, GLUTEN-FREE, NIGHTSHADE-FREE, VEGAN

SERVES 2 **PREP TIME:** 10 minutes, plus 4 hours to freeze

This delicious dairy-free ice cream is simple to make and easy to personalize with your favorite flavors. Frozen bananas provide a fiber- and antioxidant-rich base for this ice cream and the cacao powder adds flavonols to improve gut microbiome balance. Cashew milk and pecans also add healthy unsaturated fats and protein for both creaminess and crunch.

4 medium bananas, peeled, cut into chunks, and frozen

¼ cup cacao powder

2 tablespoons cashew butter

½ cup Creamy Cashew Milk (page 133)

4 tablespoons chopped pecans, divided

1. In a food processer, combine the frozen bananas, cacao powder, cashew butter, and cashew milk. Pulse until the bananas are broken into smaller chunks. Stop the processor and scrape down the sides with a spatula.

2. Process again on high speed until the mixture is creamy. Transfer the ice cream base to a freezer-safe dish and freeze for at least 4 hours.

3. When ready to serve, let the ice cream soften at room temperature for 10 minutes.

4. Top each serving with 2 tablespoons chopped pecans.

Ingredient tip: You can substitute ½ cup of any soy-based milk or other dairy-free milk for the Creamy Cashew Milk in this recipe.

Per Serving: Calories: 506; Total Fat: 24g; Saturated Fat: 4g; Cholesterol: 0mg; Carbohydrates: 72g; Fiber: 13g; Protein: 12g

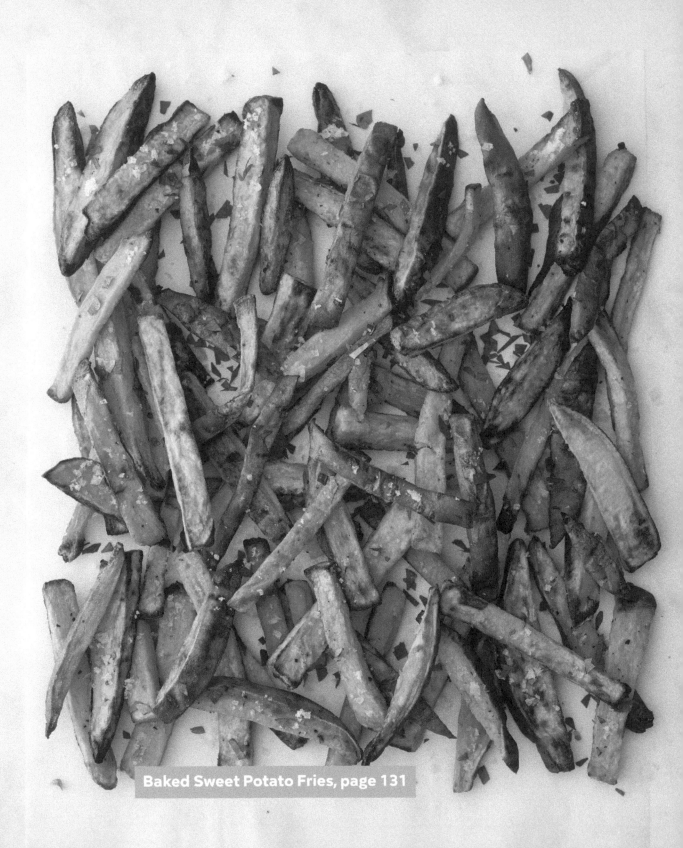

Baked Sweet Potato Fries, page 131

9
SIDES, SNACKS, AND STAPLES

Anti-Inflammatory Cauliflower Soup

DAIRY-FREE, GLUTEN-FREE, NIGHTSHADE-FREE, VEGAN
SERVES 4 **PREP TIME:** 15 minutes **COOK TIME:** 35 minutes

Cauliflower has become an anti-inflammatory superstar, and rightly so! The cruciferous vegetable is packed with vitamin C to support healthy immune system function and fiber to feed the gut. The polyphenols and sulfur-containing compounds in cauliflower also act as powerful antioxidants. Ginger and turmeric boost this soup's anti-inflammatory benefits even more. Serve as-is or pureed with an immersion blender for a creamier texture.

2 tablespoons avocado oil

1 large rutabaga, peeled and diced

1 small head cauliflower, chopped

1 small yellow onion, chopped

1 garlic clove, minced

1 tablespoon grated peeled fresh ginger

2 teaspoons ground turmeric

2 teaspoons ground coriander

1 teaspoon ground cumin

½ teaspoon sea salt

4 cups low-sodium vegetable broth

1. In a large stockpot over medium heat, heat the oil. Add the rutabaga, cauliflower, and onion and sauté for about 10 minutes, or until softened.

2. Stir in the garlic, ginger, turmeric, coriander, cumin, salt, and broth. Increase the heat to high and bring the soup to a boil. Reduce the heat to medium-low and cover the pot. Simmer for 20 minutes, until the vegetables are tender.

Batch cook tip: This soup freezes well, so double the recipe and transfer half to a freezer-safe container and keep frozen for up to 3 months. Thaw in the refrigerator overnight, then reheat in a medium saucepan over medium heat for 10 minutes.

Per Serving: Calories: 179; Total Fat: 8g; Saturated Fat: 1g; Cholesterol: 0mg; Carbohydrates: 26g; Fiber: 7g; Protein: 5g

Wilted Spinach with Chickpeas

DAIRY-FREE, GLUTEN-FREE, NIGHTSHADE-FREE, VEGAN
SERVES 4 **PREP TIME:** 10 minutes **COOK TIME:** 15 minutes

This perfect side dish gets lots of nutty flavor from chickpeas. It's also full of fiber and protein, making it a good entrée option. Phytochemicals and other bioactive compounds that help reduce oxidation and inflammation in the body come from the spinach, as does quercetin, which is important for lowering inflammation.

3 tablespoons avocado oil, divided

1 large onion, sliced

2 garlic cloves, crushed

1 teaspoon ground cumin

14 cups fresh spinach

1 (15-ounce) can chickpeas, drained and rinsed

½ teaspoon kosher salt

¼ teaspoon freshly ground black pepper

1. In a large skillet over medium heat, heat 1 tablespoon oil. Add the onion and garlic and sauté for about 5 minutes, or until the onion is softened and garlic is fragrant.

2. Stir in the cumin and sauté for another minute.

3. Add the spinach in batches and cook, stirring continuously, for about 5 minutes, or until wilted.

4. Stir in the chickpeas, the remaining 2 tablespoons oil, salt, and pepper. Cook until heated through. Immediately remove from heat and serve warm.

Variation tip: This recipe is also great with equal amounts of Swiss chard or curly kale in place of the spinach. Simply remove the chard or kale stems and coarsely chop them before adding to the skillet.

Per Serving: Calories: 226; Total Fat: 13g; Saturated Fat: 1g; Cholesterol: 0mg; Carbohydrates: 23g; Fiber: 7g; Protein: 8g

Carrot Salad with Spicy Greens

DAIRY-FREE, GLUTEN-FREE, NIGHTSHADE-FREE, VEGETARIAN
SERVES 4 **PREP TIME:** 10 minutes

Arugula is a peppery green that adds a spicy bite to any fresh salad. It also acts as a powerful antioxidant and provides a variety of minerals and vitamins. With the inclusion of apple cider vinegar, which acts as a fermented food, this salad is a great option for balancing the gut microbiome.

3 large carrots, grated

6 cups arugula, coarsely chopped

3 tablespoons extra-virgin olive oil

2 tablespoons apple cider vinegar with the mother

2 teaspoons honey

1 teaspoon freshly squeezed lemon juice

1 teaspoon dried oregano

½ teaspoon kosher salt

¼ teaspoon freshly ground black pepper

1. In a large bowl, mix the carrots and arugula.

2. In a small, lidded mason jar or salad dressing shaker, combine the oil, vinegar, honey, lemon juice, oregano, salt, and pepper. Cover the jar and shake well to blend.

3. Pour the dressing over the carrots and arugula and toss to coat.

Make it easier: If you won't be eating the whole salad, store the dressing and the salad mixture separately. Add the dressing at mealtime to avoid soggy greens.

Per Serving: Calories: 132; Total Fat: 11g; Saturated Fat: 1g; Cholesterol: 0mg; Carbohydrates: 9g; Fiber: 2g; Protein: 1g

Savory Sweet Potato Hummus

DAIRY-FREE, GLUTEN-FREE, NIGHTSHADE-FREE, VEGAN

SERVES 4 **PREP TIME:** 5 minutes **COOK TIME:** 35 minutes

This sweet potato hummus takes traditional hummus to another level. Sweet potatoes add a rich color and even more fiber to an already fiber-rich dish, as well as vitamin C and beta-carotene. The extra-virgin olive oil provides potent antioxidant and anti-inflammatory benefits. Serve this hummus with vegetable sticks, as a salad topper, or with nut crackers.

1 medium sweet potato

1 (15-ounce) can chickpeas, drained and rinsed

1 garlic clove, peeled

1½ tablespoons extra-virgin olive oil

1 tablespoon freshly squeezed lemon juice

¾ teaspoon sea salt

½ teaspoon ground cumin

¼ teaspoon ground cinnamon

1. Preheat the oven to 400°F. Line a baking sheet with parchment paper.

2. Pierce the skin of the sweet potato several times with a knife and place it on the prepared baking sheet.

3. Bake for 35 minutes, or until softened. Transfer the sweet potato to a medium bowl and mash the sweet potato with the skin on. Transfer the mashed sweet potato to a blender.

4. Add the chickpeas, garlic, oil, lemon juice, salt, cumin, and cinnamon and blend until smooth.

Ingredient tip: To save time, pierce the skin of the sweet potato and microwave it on high power for 2 to 3 minutes per side. I like to bake several sweet potatoes at once and keep them in the refrigerator for use in recipes through-out the week.

Per Serving: Calories: 168; Total Fat: 7g; Saturated Fat: 1g; Cholesterol: 0mg; Carbohydrates: 22g; Fiber: 5g; Protein: 5g

Simple Roasted Vegetables

DAIRY-FREE, GLUTEN-FREE, NIGHTSHADE-FREE, VEGAN
SERVES 4 PREP TIME: 15 minutes COOK TIME: 35 minutes

Roasted vegetables are an easy way to consume a variety of nutrients in one serving. Swap in whatever vegetables you have on hand, but this recipe uses mushrooms, daikon radish, and kohlrabi. Mushrooms have been used for centuries for their medicinal benefits and act as pre-biotics for the gut microbiome. Daikon radish is high in vitamin C to support a healthy immune system and contains powerful polyphenols to fight inflammation. Make a big batch and store leftovers in the refrigerator for up to 3 days.

2 cups cauliflower florets

1 medium yellow squash, sliced

1 medium zucchini, sliced

1 cup baby bella mushrooms, sliced

1 large carrot, cut into chunks

1 medium daikon radish, peeled and cut into chunks

1 medium kohlrabi, trimmed, peeled, and cut into chunks

¼ cup avocado oil

1 teaspoon dried oregano

1 teaspoon dried basil

½ teaspoon dried thyme

½ teaspoon sea salt

¼ teaspoon freshly ground black pepper

1. Preheat the oven to 400°F. Line a baking sheet with parchment paper.

2. In a large bowl, mix the cauliflower, squash, zucchini, mushrooms, carrot, radish, and kohlrabi well.

3. In a small bowl, whisk the oil, oregano, basil, thyme, salt, and pepper to combine. Pour the dressing over the vegetables and toss to coat. Spread the vegetables on the prepared baking sheet.

4. Roast for 35 minutes, or until tender.

Ingredient tip: Kohlrabi is a cruciferous vegetable available in most grocery stores. It has a mild cabbage-like flavor and can be roasted, sautéed, and eaten raw in salads. Kohlrabi greens can also be added to green smoothies.

Per Serving: Calories: 189; Total Fat: 14g; Saturated Fat: 2g; Cholesterol: 0mg; Carbohydrates: 14g; Fiber: 6g; Protein: 4g

Pumpkin Seed Butter

DAIRY-FREE, GLUTEN-FREE, NIGHTSHADE-FREE, VEGAN

MAKES 1½ cups **PREP TIME:** 10 minutes **COOK TIME:** 5 minutes, plus 10 minutes to cool

Despite the bad rap that nuts and seeds sometimes get due to their high calorie and fat content, they're full of anti-inflammatory unsaturated fats and have antioxidants as well as minerals, such as selenium and magnesium—often lacking in the American diet. Because many premade nut and seed butters found in the grocery store have inflammatory oils and sugar added, making your own nut and seed butters is a great way to save money and avoid those inflammatory ingredients.

1 cup raw pepitas (shelled pumpkin seeds)	½ cup whole shelled hemp seeds	¼ teaspoon ground nutmeg
1 cup raw sunflower seeds	1 tablespoon chia seeds	¼ teaspoon sea salt
¼ cup raw cashews	1 tablespoon ground cinnamon	¼ cup coconut oil

1. Preheat the oven to 325°F. Line a baking sheet with parchment paper.

2. Spread the pepitas, sunflower seeds, and cashews on the prepared baking sheet.

3. Roast for 5 minutes, or until the cashews are lightly browned. Let the roasted seeds and cashews cool for 10 minutes.

4. In a food processor or blender, combine the roasted and cooled seed and nut mix, hemp seeds, chia seeds, cinnamon, nutmeg, salt, and coconut oil. Blend on high speed to form a smooth, spreadable consistency. (This may take several minutes.)

Ingredient tip: This seed butter lasts for up to 1 month in a tightly sealed container in the refrigerator. Add 1 tablespoon to green smoothies or enjoy the butter with fresh fruit slices.

Per Serving: (2 tablespoons) Calories: 227; Total Fat: 20g; Saturated Fat: 6g;

Cholesterol: 0mg; Carbohydrates: 6g; Fiber: 3g; Protein: 8g

Roasted Cauliflower "Steaks"

DAIRY-FREE, GLUTEN-FREE, NIGHTSHADE-FREE, VEGAN

SERVES 4 **PREP TIME:** 10 minutes **COOK TIME:** 25 minutes

Cauliflower is a versatile vegetable. It also packs a nutritional punch. It is high in fiber to fuel the gut microbiome, and it provides a significant source of vitamin C to maintain a healthy immune system. Like its cruciferous cousins, cauliflower contains the powerful antioxidant sulforaphane, which is important for cancer prevention and treatment.

2 large cauliflower heads

¼ cup avocado oil

1 tablespoon freshly squeezed lemon juice

¾ teaspoon garlic powder

¾ teaspoon sea salt

½ teaspoon freshly ground black pepper

½ teaspoon dried thyme

1. Preheat the oven to 450°F. Line a baking sheet with parchment paper.

2. Halve the two cauliflower heads down the center and slice a 1-inch "steak" from each of the four halves. Place the cauliflower steaks on the prepared baking sheet. Chop the remaining cauliflower and refrigerate it in an airtight container for another use, such as a side dish or in a salad.

3. In a small bowl, whisk the oil, lemon juice, garlic powder, salt, pepper, and thyme to blend. Using half the dressing, brush each cauliflower steak.

4. Bake for 12 minutes. Turn the cauliflower steaks over and brush each with the remaining dressing. Bake for 12 minutes more, until lightly browned and tender.

Variation tip: Create a slightly different flavor by using a combination of ½ teaspoon of dried oregano, ½ teaspoon of dried basil, and ¾ teaspoon of onion powder in place of the garlic powder and thyme.

Per Serving: Calories: 229; Total Fat: 15g; Saturated Fat: 2g; Cholesterol: 0mg; Carbohydrates: 22g; Fiber: 9g; Protein: 8g

Garlic Brussels Sprouts

DAIRY-FREE, GLUTEN-FREE, NIGHTSHADE-FREE, VEGAN

SERVES 4 **PREP TIME:** 5 minutes **COOK TIME:** 15 minutes

Brussels sprouts don't smell great while cooking, but the finished product is so worth it. A member of the cruciferous family, Brussels sprouts contain vitamin C for immune system function, vitamin K for blood clotting, and fiber to fuel the gut microbiome. With the added health benefits of garlic, this recipe makes a powerful inflammation-fighting side dish.

1 teaspoon extra-virgin olive oil

¼ cup sliced yellow onion

6 garlic cloves, minced

1 pound Brussels sprouts, trimmed (see tip) and thinly sliced

½ teaspoon sea salt

¼ teaspoon freshly ground black pepper

1. In a large stainless-steel or cast-iron skillet over medium heat, heat the oil. Add the onion and sauté for about 3 minutes, or until fragrant.

2. Add the garlic and sauté for 1 minute.

3. Add the Brussels sprouts, salt, and pepper and sauté for about 10 minutes, or until the vegetables are browned.

Ingredient tip: Brussels sprouts can be bought fresh in bags, whole on the stalk, or frozen. If using fresh Brussels sprouts, trim away the brown area where they were originally connected to the stalk (unless you've just removed them from the stalk).

Per Serving: Calories: 70; Total Fat: 2g; Saturated Fat: <1g; Cholesterol: 0mg; Carbohydrates: 13g; Fiber: 5g; Protein: 4g

Fresh Guacamole

DAIRY-FREE, GLUTEN-FREE, VEGAN

SERVES 4 PREP TIME: 10 minutes

Avocados are packed with fiber and healthy monounsaturated fat to fuel healthy metabolism and decrease inflammation. People who eat avocados tend to have higher intakes of fiber, vitamins E and K, and the minerals magnesium and potassium. Eating avocados regularly leads to better cardiovascular health and may promote healthy aging and healthy weight management. What better way to take advantage of all these benefits than with guacamole?

2 garlic cloves, minced

¼ cup minced red onion

¼ jalapeño pepper, minced

2 avocados, peeled, halved, and pitted

1 tablespoon freshly squeezed lime juice

½ teaspoon ground coriander

¼ teaspoon sea salt

1. In a medium bowl, stir together the garlic, red onion, and jalapeno.

2. Add the avocado and mash the ingredients well with a fork.

3. Stir in the lime juice, coriander, and salt.

Ingredient tip: Guacamole can brown quickly. To keep it fresher longer, keep the avocado pit and place it in the guacamole mixture while storing, covered, in the refrigerator.

Per Serving: Calories: 122; Total Fat: 11g; Saturated Fat: 2g; Cholesterol: 0mg; Carbohydrates: 8g; Fiber: 5g; Protein: 2g

Baked Sweet Potato Fries

DAIRY-FREE, GLUTEN-FREE, NIGHTSHADE-FREE, VEGAN

SERVES 4 **PREP TIME:** 5 minutes **COOK TIME:** 45 minutes

French fries are a favorite American food, but white potatoes can cause inflammation for those who don't tolerate nightshades. Instead of giving up fries altogether, try this healthy alternative using sweet potatoes. Sweet potatoes are much more nutritionally dense and provide valuable beta-carotene, fiber, potassium, and vitamin C.

4 medium sweet potatoes, cut into ¼-inch strips

2 tablespoons avocado oil

2 teaspoons dried oregano

½ teaspoon sea salt

½ teaspoon freshly ground black pepper

1. Preheat the oven to 400°F. Line a baking sheet with parchment paper.

2. In a large bowl, combine the sweet potato strips, oil, oregano, salt, and pepper. Toss to coat the sweet potatoes. Spread the sweet potatoes in a single layer on the prepared baking sheet.

3. Bake for 45 minutes, or until the sweet potatoes are golden brown and crispy, stirring every 15 minutes.

Ingredient tip: To maximize nutrient intake, keep the skin on the sweet potatoes.

Per Serving: Calories: 173; Total Fat: 7g; Saturated Fat: 1g; Cholesterol: 0mg; Carbohydrates: 27g; Fiber: 4g; Protein: 2g

Simple Italian Salad Dressing

DAIRY-FREE, GLUTEN-FREE, NIGHTSHADE-FREE, VEGAN

MAKES about ¾ cup **PREP TIME:** 10 minutes

Extra-virgin olive oil is a staple in the Mediterranean diet—and for good reason. This mostly monounsaturated fat has been shown to reduce the risk of cardiovascular disease, type 2 diabetes, and obesity. Olive oil also contains phenolic compounds that have antioxidant and anti-inflammatory properties, making it an inflammation-fighting powerhouse. Made with apple cider vinegar, this tangy dressing jazzes up any salad.

½ cup extra-virgin olive oil

¼ cup apple cider vinegar with the mother

1 tablespoon Dijon mustard

2 garlic cloves, minced

1 tablespoon Italian seasoning

¼ teaspoon sea salt

⅛ teaspoon freshly ground black pepper

In a small, lidded mason jar or salad dressing shaker, combine the oil, vinegar, mustard, garlic, Italian seasoning, salt, and pepper. Cover the jar and shake well to combine.

Variation tip: For a little sweetness, add 2 teaspoons of pure maple syrup to the dressing.

Per Serving: (2 tablespoons) Calories: 250; Total Fat: 27g; Saturated Fat: 4g; Cholesterol: 0mg; Carbohydrates: 1g; Fiber: 1g; Protein: <1g

Creamy Cashew Milk

DAIRY-FREE, GLUTEN-FREE, NIGHTSHADE-FREE, VEGAN

MAKES about 4 cups PREP TIME: 10 minutes, plus 15 minutes to soak

Store-bought nut milks often contain additives, sugar, and other ingredients that can be inflammatory. They are also lower in certain nutrients. Homemade cashew milk is higher in plant-based protein and anti-inflammatory fats. Cashews are also high in copper, which is an important mineral for maintaining overall skin health.

1 cup raw cashews

6 cups hot water, divided

1 tablespoon pure maple syrup

⅛ teaspoon sea salt

1. In a small bowl, combine the cashews and 2 cups hot water. Let soak for 15 minutes. Drain the cashews and discard the soaking water.

2. In a blender, combine the soaked cashews, maple syrup, salt, and the remaining 4 cups hot water. Blend on high speed for about 2 minutes, until creamy.

3. Transfer the cashew milk to an airtight storage jar (no need to strain) and refrigerate for up to 5 days.

Batch cook tip: Cashew milk can be used in a variety of recipes, so double the recipe to save time later in the week.

Per Serving: (1 cup) Calories: 193; Total Fat: 14g; Saturated Fat: 3g; Cholesterol: 0mg; Carbohydrates: 13g; Fiber: 1g; Protein: 6g

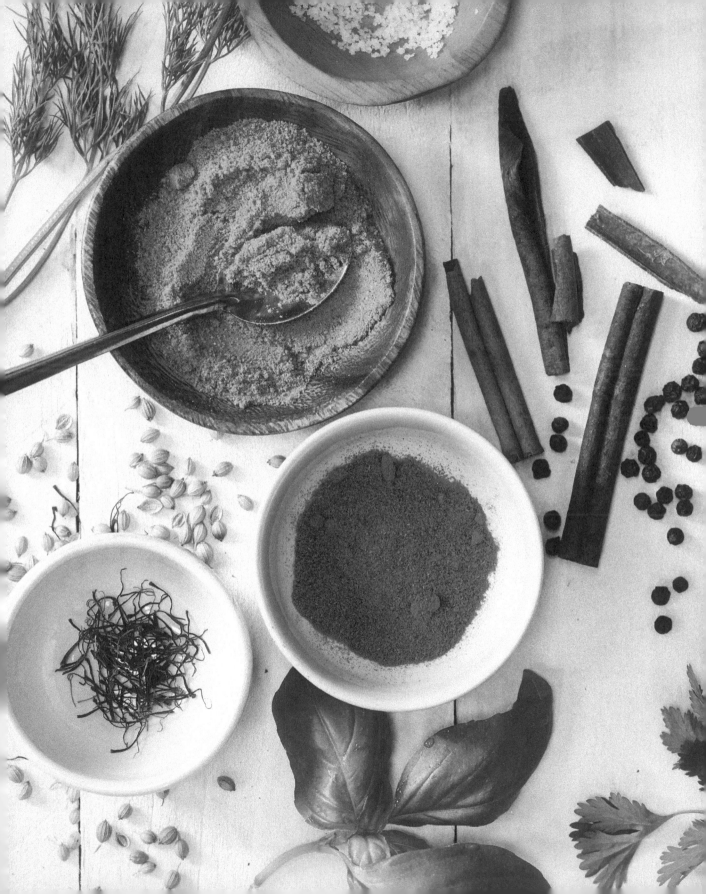

MEASUREMENT CONVERSIONS

	U.S. STANDARD	U.S. STANDARD (OUNCES)	METRIC (APPROXIMATE)
VOLUME EQUIVALENTS (LIQUID)	2 tablespoons	1 fl. oz.	30 mL
	¼ cup	2 fl. oz.	60 mL
	½ cup	4 fl. oz.	120 mL
	1 cup	8 fl. oz.	240 mL
	1½ cups	12 fl. oz.	355 mL
	2 cups or 1 pint	16 fl. oz.	475 mL
	4 cups or 1 quart	32 fl. oz.	1 L
	1 gallon	128 fl. oz.	4 L
VOLUME EQUIVALENTS (DRY)	teaspoon	————	0.5 mL
	¼ teaspoon	————	1 mL
	½ teaspoon	————	2 mL
	¾ teaspoon	————	4 mL
	1 teaspoon	————	5 mL
	1 tablespoon	————	15 mL
	¼ cup	————	59 mL
	cup	————	79 mL
	½ cup	————	118 mL
	cup	————	156 mL
	¾ cup	————	177 mL
	1 cup	————	235 mL
	2 cups or 1 pint	————	475 mL
	3 cups	————	700 mL
	4 cups or 1 quart	————	1 L
	½ gallon	————	2 L
	1 gallon	————	4 L
WEIGHT EQUIVALENTS	½ ounce	————	15 g
	1 ounce	————	30 g
	2 ounces	————	60 g
	4 ounces	————	115 g
	8 ounces	————	225 g
	12 ounces	————	340 g
	16 ounces or 1 pound	————	455 g

	FAHRENHEIT (F)	CELSIUS (C) (APPROXIMATE)
OVEN TEMPERATURES	250°F	120°C
	300°F	150°C
	325°F	180°C
	375°F	190°C
	400°F	200°C
	425°F	220°C
	450°F	230°C

RESOURCES

Websites

Local Harvest (LocalHarvest.org): Website dedicated to connecting consumers with local farmers.

Monterey Bay Aquarium Seafood Watch (SeafoodWatch.org): Website dedicated to educating consumers about sustainable seafood.

National Library of Medicine (Pubmed.NCBI.NLM.NIH.gov): Website providing the latest research trials.

National Psoriasis Foundation (Psoriasis.org): Website dedicated to psoriasis treatment. Contains research trial information and the latest psoriasis treatment options.

NutriSense Nutrition Consulting, LLC (NutriSenseNutrition.com): My blog and website offers functional nutrition information for anyone looking to prevent or reverse chronic disease. You can read more about my personal story, recipes, and ways to improve your quality of life with lifestyle- and nutrition-related strategies.

The American Academy of Dermatology (AAD.org): Website providing resources for all skin-related conditions.

The Institute for Functional Medicine (IFM.org): Website providing information about functional medicine and a tool for finding a functional medicine practitioner.

Books

Gluten Freedom: The Nation's Leading Expert Offers the Essential Guide to a Healthy Gluten-Free Lifestyle by Alessio Fasano, MD and Susie Flaherty (New York: John Wiley & Sons, 2014).

Missing Microbes: How the Overuse of Antibiotics Is Fueling Our Modern Plagues by Martin J. Blaser, MD (London: Picador, 2014).

The Autoimmune Solution: Prevent and Reverse the Full Spectrum of Inflammatory Symptoms and Disease by Amy Myers, MD. (New York: HarperOne, 2017).

The Psoriasis Diet Cookbook: Easy, Healthy Recipes to Soothe Your Symptoms by Kellie Blake, RDN, LD, IFNCP (Emeryville, CA: Rockridge Press, 2020).

REFERENCES

Bronckers, I. M., A. S. Paller, M. J. van Geel, P. C. van de Kerkhof, and M. M. Seyger. "Psoriasis in Children and Adolescents: Diagnosis, Management and Comorbidities." *Paediatric Drugs 17*, no. 5 (2015): 373–384. doi.org/10.1007/s40272-015-0137-1.

Clemente, J. C., J. Manasson, and J. U. Scher. "The Role of the Gut Microbiome in Systemic Inflammatory Disease." *British Medical Journal (clinical research ed.;* 2018). Retrieved from: https://pubmed.ncbi.nlm.nih.gov/29311119/.

De Santis, S., M. Cariello, E. Piccinin, C. Sabbà, and A. Moschetta. "Extra-Virgin Olive Oil: Lesson from Nutrigenomics." *Nutrients 11*, no. 9 (2019): 2085. doi.org/10.3390/nu11092085.

Dimidi, E., S. R. Cox, M. Rossi, and K. Whelan. "Fermented Foods: Definitions and Characteristics: Impact on the Gut Microbiota and Effects on Gastrointestinal Health and Disease." *Nutrients 11, no.* 8 (2019): 1806. doi.org/10.3390/nu11081806.

Fasano A. (2020). "All Disease Begins in the (Leaky) Gut: Role of Zonulin-Mediated Gut Permeability in the Pathogenesis of Some Chronic Inflammatory Diseases." *F1000Research 9*, F1000 Faculty Rev-69. doi.org/10.12688/f1000research.20510.1

Kamiya, K., M. Kishimoto, J. Sugai, M. Komine, and M. Ohtsuki. "Risk Factors for the Development of Psoriasis." *International Journal of Molecular Sciences 20*, no. 18 (2019): 4347. doi.org/10.3390/ijms20184347.

Khan, N., and H. Mukhtar. "Tea Polyphenols in Promotion of Human Health." *Nutrients 11*, no. 1 (2018): 39. doi.org/10.3390/nu11010039.

Menter, A. "Psoriasis and Psoriatic Arthritis Overview." *The American Journal of Managed Care 22*, no. 8 Supplement (2016): s216–s224.

Musial, C., A. Kuban-Jankowska, and M. Gorska-Ponikowska. "Beneficial Properties of Green Tea Catechins." *International Journal of Molecular Sciences 21*, no. 5 (2020): 1744. doi.org/10.3390/ijms21051744.

Paoli, A., L. Mancin, A. Bianco, E. Thomas, J. F. Mota, and F. Piccini. "Ketogenic Diet and Microbiota: Friends or Enemies?" *Genes 10*, no. 7 (2019): 534. doi.org/10.3390/genes10070534.

Rendon, A., and K. Schäkel. "Psoriasis Pathogenesis and Treatment." *International Journal of Molecular Sciences 20*, no. 6 (2019): 1475. doi.org/10.3390/ijms20061475.

Wang, Q. P., D. Browman, H. Herzog, and G. G. Neely. "Non-Nutritive Sweeteners Possess a Bacteriostatic Effect and Alter Gut Microbiota in Mice." *PLoS ONE 13*, no. 7 (2018): e0199080. doi.org/10.1371/journal.pone.0199080.

INDEX

ACKNOWLEDGMENTS

I am truly blessed with so much support from my family and friends. I want to especially acknowledge my husband, Will, who has changed his entire lifestyle to support my health mission. When I started on this journey four years ago, it would have been a million times harder had he not been there by my side, encouraging me. He didn't ask questions or complain about having to change. Instead, he just jumped on the healthy train with me and asked how he could help. He is always there to make me laugh, taste new recipes, and, when it's his turn to make dinner, he's a pro!

And thank you to the entire Callisto team for giving me another opportunity to share the food-as-medicine message.

ABOUT THE AUTHOR

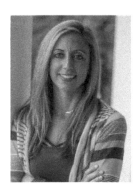

Kellie Blake, RDN, LD, IFNCP, is a registered dietitian specializing in functional nutrition. Kellie works in a variety of settings including psychiatry, hospice, and enteral nutrition. She co-owns a private practice, NutriSense Nutrition Consulting, LLC, where she determines the root causes of her clients' symptoms and uses a functional nutrition approach to help them regain their health and quality of life. Kellie is also the chief nutrition officer of KyKana Corporation, a Kentucky-based company on a mission to provide healing in Appalachia. Kellie is a health and nutrition writer. She currently serves on the editorial board of Integrative Practitioner, where she writes monthly articles highlighting her client case studies. Find Kellie on NutriSenseNutrition.com or on Instagram @NutriSenseNutrition.